"Transient are all conditioned things.

Work out your salvation with diligence."

Last Words of Gautama the Buddha

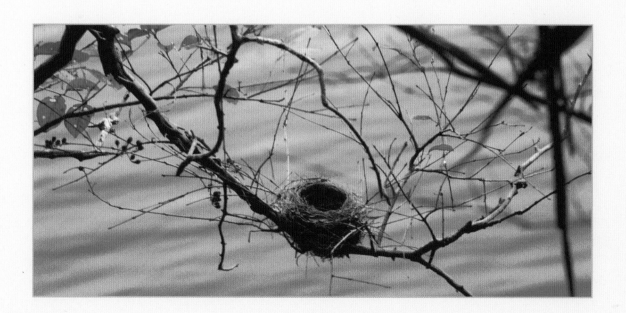

Managing Expectations & Comparisons

A Guide to Go Beyond Stress

Athmo

with all my love

to

you

from

Athmo

..

Moksha Publications

This Book is Dedicated to

Osho for being there and getting me started. A thousand thanks. The entire Enlow family: especially Ellsworth Enlow (Grandpa). All the Rishis, Munis, Yogis, Sadhus, Monks and anybody on the path of self-discovery.

A Thousand Thanks

My mother (Sudershana) for her helping with everyday needs and being there. Rita Enlow (Sunder) for being there every step of the way. Katheryn Seman (Misha) and Anila Manning for spending lots of hours editing the book and enjoying it as much as I did. Prem Sarita for all our experiences that helped me to see the next step. This book would not be possible without the strong support of my friends, family and all my students.

A Special Thanks

To Ilana Peled of Tel Aviv, Israel for all the incredible photographs of flowers and nature. This book would not be complete and beautiful without her contributions. You can see all of her work at: http://www.ilanapeled.com.

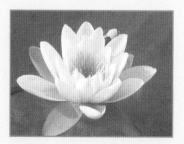

Contents

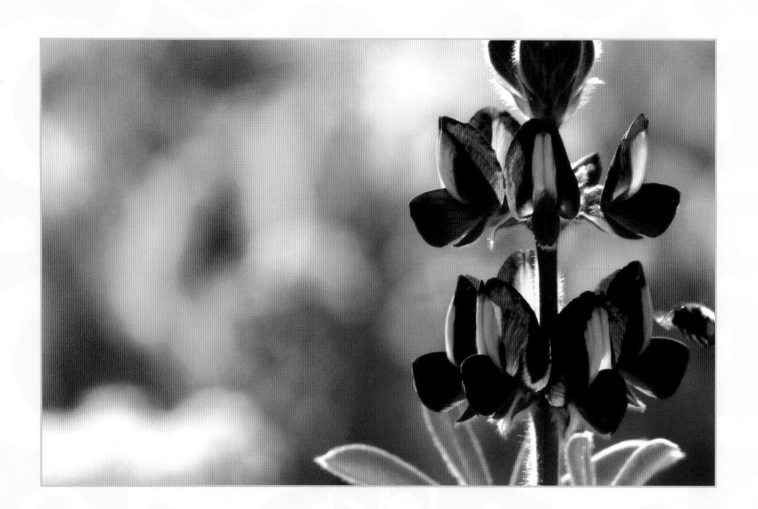

In the pursuit of learning,
every day something is acquired.

In the pursuit of Tao,
every day something is dropped.

Less and less is done,
Until non-action is achieved.

When nothing is done,
nothing is left undone.

The world is ruled by letting things take their course;
It cannot be ruled by interfering.

Lao Tsu, Tao Te Ching Forty-Eight

Why This Book?

A recent comprehensive European study which followed 25,000 people in 52 countries, and took a decade to complete concluded that stress is the number one predictor of cardiovascular disease or a heart attack. Specifically the study found that psychosocial stress such as stress at work and at home, financial stress, and major life events in the past year were extremely significant in predicting heart attacks. Heart attack is the number one killer in the world today. The numbers are so staggering that the medical experts are equating this problem to the "Black Death" from the middle ages that killed over half the population of the world in under two years. Unfortunately, there is very little that we know about how to cope with or eliminate stress. Stress is a vast phenomenon that can happen in short period of time without any warning. Our medical treatment for stress today is often some type of medication that can have severe side effects.

What is Stress?

Stress is the difference between what is and what is expected.

This definition of stress has two components: what is and what is expected. If in a given situation "what is" and "what is expected" are hard to determine then your stress is going to be very high. For example; if you are assigned a job that does not state exactly what is required of you, but you are asked to fulfill unclear expectations, then you will have a lot of stress. This is because you don't know what the job entails and the expectations are unclear.

Having no stress means having a balance between "what is" and "what is expected."

This balance can only be achieved if one becomes totally conscious in whatever one does. Unfortunately, we live our lives in a very unconscious way. For example, Imagine you are reading a book and suddenly (as always) a thought enters your consciousness and engages you. You will probably continue to keep reading while you are also engaged with the thought and therefore be unable to comprehend anything. If you are reading the book for a test next day you are going to be stressed because you are unable to comprehend. This is because your expectation is to comprehend the material in a reasonable period of time and the reality is that is not happening.

If your consciousness is undisturbed by any outside thoughts you will find that reading the material once will be enough for you to comprehend the material. This is the goal of this book: to share with you techniques that will remove the disturbance from your consciousness. This will help you to do things efficiently without repeating the acts needlessly and stressing yourself.

As you practice the exercises discussed in the book you will be able to determine the two components of stress right away: "what is" and "what is expected." As you practice remaining totally conscious in whatever you do your attention will be focused without any disturbance.

In such a situation it will be easy to determine "what is." Once you are clear about what is required you will be able to know which expectations can be fulfilled and which cannot. This will help you to be clear about your and other people's expectations upon you. If particular expectations cannot be met your decision will be clear to you. This will help you to steer away from stress at all times and avoid any unnecessary suffering to your body or consciousness. Consciousness is like a light that you bring into your mind (dark room). It makes it easy for you to move around and do things which would be otherwise difficult.

Nothing is assumed about you. If you are interested in silence, relaxation and how to de-stress your consciousness and body, this is definitely your book. Yoga and Qi-gong exercises are used for relaxation, but they have no religious affiliations (you don't have to be Hindu or Buddhist to practice them). Yoga exercises will stretch your body and relax it while Qi-gong exercises will circulate the

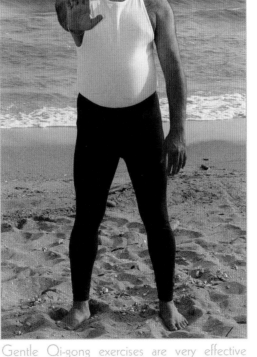

Gentle Qi-gong exercises are very effective in letting the consciousness flow through your body.

energy and bring you to a state of oneness. You can think of them as the chisel and hammer that you need to make a beautiful sculpture. Your chisel is the yoga, your hammer is the Qi-gong and the beautiful sculpture is you in your body. Neither tool is more important; you cannot think of one without the other.

The book is hands-on. Each chapter introduces ideas and techniques, followed by exercises so you can experience their effects and not just know them theoretically. I suggest that you read each chapter a few times and then do the exercises. After a few days of practice, come back, read the material again and see how your experiences have deepened. Doing the exercises will tune your body to the frequency of consciousness. Your experiences will then be similar to what the book describes.

Thanks for reading and giving me an opportunity to be with you.

Athmo

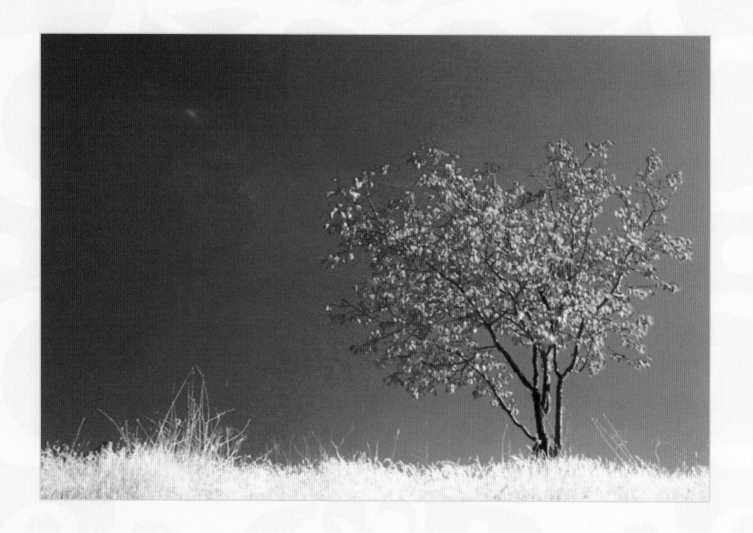

तत् उपराग अपेक्षितत्वात् चित्तस्य वस्तु ज्ञात अज्ञातम्

Tat uparaaga apekshitattvaat cittasya vastu jnata ajnatam.

An object remains known or unknown according to the
conditioning or expectations in the consciousness.

Patanjali, Yoga Sutras, Kevalya Pada, IV-17

Imagine you and your best friend are having a conversation. Every two minutes someone else is interrupting with questions. Each time you are interrupted, you find it is hard to continue from where you left off. In the end, you may not even remember what the conversation was about. You were both involved in so many other conversations that the conversation you wanted to have was never completed. If you are alert to this phenomenon, you will immediately say, "Let's have our conversation where nobody will disturb us."

In our minds, this is what happens all day long. You would like to focus on and complete one thing, but other thoughts in the form of chatter always come in the way of what you are trying to do. It is interesting to notice that when you try to be quiet or relax, even more stray thoughts come into your consciousness. If you don't relax or find quiet times in your life, these unrelated thoughts are there anyway. Unfortunately, we don't know how it should be or how many or which types of thoughts we should have when we are doing a particular task.

Let us say you are going to make lemonade. If you have never made lemonade before, you will need the correct ingredients and concise directions. If the directions are not clear, or if the ingredients are mixed in a box with other unrelated food items, you will have a hard time making it. You will spend more time guessing and finding the right things to make lemonade. Without clarity, if it is hard to make a simple thing like lemonade how difficult would it be to make a gourmet dish where there are more steps involved and several precisely-measured ingredients?

Your ability to see clearly what a task requires and organize the ingredients and the information needed is going to be key in successfully completing it. If you are organized, you will find that you are also able to become creative in doing things. For example, you might want to make different flavors of lemonade. Creativity is the growth that we all seek in whatever we do. If we lack creativity, we often feel stuck and give up.

Take a moment, think, and make a list of all things that you enjoy and feel that you are very good at. You will find one or all of the following:

- While doing the task you are able to focus easily.
- You are very organized while doing the task.
- You can easily tell the difference between relevant and irrelevant information.
- You enjoy what you are doing so much that you forget everything else, even the time.
- Above all, you are extremely conscious while doing the task.

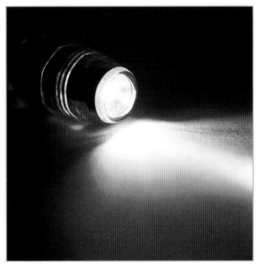

Consciousness and Light

In anything that you do, your level of consciousness is going to be the only deciding factor for how efficiently you complete a given task. For example, if you have one intoxicated and one sober person making lemonade, the intoxicated one will probably have a hard time putting ingredients together, while the clear and sober person will be able to complete the task with ease and explain what they did. Consciousness is like a light that you have so you can see things before you take any action. If you have no consciousness, or a disturbed consciousness, then it is like working with poor or no light at all.

Imagine you enter an unfamiliar, dark room. The first thing you want to do is find a light source. In the absence of that, your mobility will greatly be restricted and there is the fear that you might get injured or physically harmed by your movement in the room. Once you realize that it is too dangerous to be in this room, you get out of it, find a flashlight, and re-enter the room. This time there is a significant difference in your confidence, movement and ability to do things that you could not do before. You discover a switch connected to a light bulb, turn the switch on and fill the room with light. Now your whole perspective of the room changes. Things that you had assumed before are instantaneously corrected. Your fears subside and you move around the room with ease and agility.

This analogy can be applied to a human being. The dark room is your body. The light source, either a flashlight or a light bulb is your level of consciousness. Your efficiency or effectiveness in being in this dark room depends upon what type of a light source you have access to. With a 1-watt flashlight, very little of the room will be revealed to you at a time. However, with a 1000-watt light bulb, you will be able to see it all at once and will not have to put the parts together in your head.

The consciousness that you experience in your body can either function as a flashlight or as a light bulb. When it functions as a flashlight, it is so narrow and weak due to the weight of the mind that it can barely illuminate anything and it moves so erratically that almost nothing can be comprehended. When we can see only a small portion of reality at any time, we become fixated and think that we are only that narrow band of light, the "individual consciousness." When the electricity (or energy, or spirit) flows correctly through the body it radiates all 1000 watts and we melt into the balanced calm and clarity of "universal consciousness."

Without exception, human beings have an innate desire to transform their flashlights into light bulbs. In our own ways, we seek this transformation all our lives. How concentrated your efforts are and how well you understand the body and its mysterious workings will determine your success.

Flashlight and Light Bulb

If you want to see something in a dark room and you only have a flashlight, you will have to focus it in the direction of your interest. This is like our concentration: When we concentrate, we focus all our consciousness in one direction. However, you will notice that when you focus only in one direction, everything else will be in total darkness. Then you move the flashlight and focus it in the next direction and so on. How well you can focus will depend upon how long you are able to keep your flashlight steady. If your flashlight moves from one direction to another in split seconds, you will not be able to integrate all the information that you have seen. Similarly, if your consciousness is working like a flashlight in constant motion, then your ability to see or comprehend is going to be very limited. Without comprehension and experience, you will feel a sense of anxiety, depression and emptiness in your life.

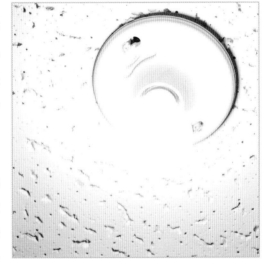

to see things clearly and you won't have to focus on them one item at a time. You will be able to comprehend what comes into and leaves your consciousness instantaneously, without straining.

This book is about how to transform your flashlight into a 100,000-watt bulb. The first five chapters focus on what causes our consciousness to behave like a flashlight and what can be done to change it into a powerful light bulb that illuminates everything. When references are made to stress, mind or chatter, they imply that your consciousness is working like a flashlight. When references are made to relaxation, alertness, and oneness, they imply that your consciousness is functioning as a light bulb. By the end, you will have an understanding that will help your consciousness remain and function only as a light bulb, and not switch back and forth from light bulb to flashlight.

When the consciousness within your body starts to function as a 1000-watt light bulb you will start

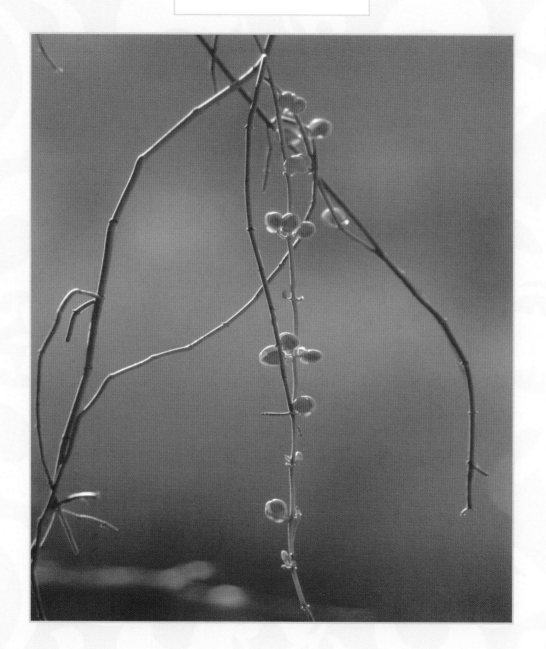

कर्मण्येवाऽधिकारस्ते मा फलेषु कदाचन

मा कर्मफलहेतुर्भूः मा ते संगोऽस्त्वकर्मणि
sansskrit

Karmani eva adhikarah te ma phaleshu kadachana
  Ma karma-phalahetuh bhuh ma te sangah astu akarmani.

Your right is for action alone, never for the results.
  Do not become the agent of the results of action.
  May you not have any inclination for inaction.

Bhagavad Gita 2.47

All desktop computers have two things: hardware and software. The hardware is the physical computer itself: computer box (CPU), monitor, mouse and keyboard. The software is a set of codes that a computer can understand to perform your desired task; this includes an operating system, office package, Internet software and any other software packages.

Similarly, a human body can be thought of as a biomechanical supercomputer that is formed by connecting several computers. Each part of the body, such as the stomach, liver, heart, or intestines can be thought of as a sub-system or sub-computer in a network of computers. The illustration shows how the stomach, liver, pancreas, small and large intestines are linked together.

A circular network exists between all the digestive organs in the body—this is how we are internally interconnected.

The human body, viewed as a computer system, has both hardware and software. The physical body is the hardware and all the learning that we have done since we were born is the software. We come with the software for basic learning. All our life we install and delete software from our brain and body; how to eat or fall in love, what religion to follow, who to marry, and how to cope with stress. If the software you have installed crashes every so often, it makes your life hard to live. Depression, anxiety and stress are results of a crash of software or hardware or both. Psychologists are programmers of human behavior and they call this programming phenomenon "conditioning." They work with different techniques to reprogram or deprogram your behavior so that you can function in a predetermined way.

Two computers cannot work together if they have conflicting software systems, and two people with different conditionings have the same problem. People with different values, religions, upbringings and languages may face a lot of difficulties in making a connection. The stronger the conditioning, the more irreconcilable the differences. A collective word for all of your conditioning (software) is "mind."

Impact of Viruses

Every computer user is aware of viruses. We spend billions of dollars on network and computer security. If a virus makes its way into the core of your computer, it can destroy your entire work, which can be equivalent to the death of your computer. Once again the same is true in your life. Viruses (disease) can take many forms impacting both your psychology and your physiology. Psychological viruses can be negative thoughts, emotions, or feelings that are destructive to your immune system and everyday functioning in life. Physiological viruses are the ones that impact your body directly such as flu, cold, HIV, hepatitis, and other infections.

The key to solving any problem is understanding and diagnosing it correctly. A whole area of computer security specializes in finding antidotes to computer viruses. This requires a thorough understanding of the computer system and the way the virus is impacting its performance. Once the virus file is clearly identified, it can be removed. In addition, any savvy computer user will use great care not to expose themselves to such viruses: by not opening attachments or messages that are infected, installing anti-virus software, installing fire-walls and filters, updating your computer system, listening and adhering to virus alerts.

The process of removing a virus (disease) is not as simple in human beings because we don't understand our bodies completely. Unlike the computer, each individual case is different because of a unique combination of psychology and physiology. The following illustration shows the functional relationship between different systems and processes in the body. It is not hard to imagine that when a disease impacts one system, it also impacts the performance of another system very quickly. For example, when you have a simple viral infection, your eyes may water, your lungs and

Der Mensch als Industriepalast

Our body is a cooperative whose survival and efficiency is interdependent upon a harmonious relationship between different organs of the body. This illustration "Der Mensch als Industriepalast" (Man as Industrial Palace) was created by Fritz Kahn. Source: National Library of Medicine sinuses may feel congested, you may have a headache, body-ache or be unable to function. Our body is a cooperative whose survival and efficiency is interdependent upon a harmonious relationship between different organs of the body.

What Do We Need to Do?

We, individually, need to take the time to understand our own body systems. We wait for our doctors to tell us what is wrong with us and many times, we don't even do that. The bottom line is that you need to be involved with your body. It is like gardening; if you have a garden and don't tend to it, weeds will grow, garbage will accumulate, and you will not have much of a garden. Your body is like your garden; if you let garbage and weeds in the form of viruses and diseases accumulate, it is going to be painful. Your body needs every-day, every-minute care. This awareness will help you to see the impact of every little thing that is happening in your life. You will be both preventive and proactive. Then it will be difficult to have a disease. You will know exactly where the system is breaking down and help in becoming a part of the solution so that you will not just be a victim of some unknown disease. You will find that the solutions are very simple; it's being able to follow through with them that is the problem.

The things that you do are a function of what you experience, learn and know. You continue or discontinue doing things depending upon what your experiences are with respect to your expectations. This learning will be the software that your body is going to use over and over again when it needs to fulfill a certain function.

Programming with Expectations & Comparisons

Our mind uses two functions: expectation and comparison. In anything we do, unconsciously or consciously, our expectation is the first thing that we define. Expectations are predetermined outcomes that you are looking for in any act or event. It is the objective function that you are trying to maximize or minimize. If you are doing business you expect to earn a certain amount of money, or in a relationship you try to minimize misunderstandings. Sometimes expectations are clearly stated, other times they can be vague and unclear. Expectation is an unwritten law that we all follow. In very rare instances in life, we do things without expectations.

Two Processes of Your Mind: Expectations and Comparisons.

When we first go to school, we are expected not to disturb anybody. If we cause a disruption, we are told what not to do and are taught accordingly. There is no clear indication given to us; we are supposed to look at what others are doing and learn from them. When we do things that the majority of people don't do, then we are out of line; we are expected to follow the norm. Teachers use rewards and punishments as tools.

There are rules that are laid out about what you are expected to do and what you are not. We use

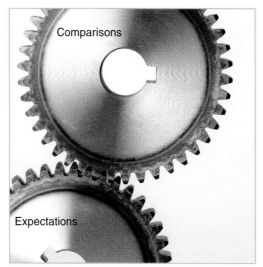

Two processes of your mind: Expectations and Comparisons

comparison to learn and fulfill things that are expected of us. Expectations and comparisons work like the thermostat on an iron. Based on the type of cloth, you are expected to set the right temperature on your iron. Once you set the temperature, the thermostat inside the iron compares the set temperature to the temperature of the iron. It starts and shuts off the heating element to meet the temperature that you are expecting. Comparison by definition requires that we compare ourselves against others at all times.

Expectations can also be thought of as goals or roles assigned to you so that you start to behave in a certain predetermined way. If you don't understand clearly what is expected of you, or if you cannot effectively compare yourself with others, you are going to be in trouble.

Expectation and comparison are two sides of the same coin; they work together in a loop. With comparison, you keep evaluating your actions and determining how close or far you are from your expectations (goal). Unfortunately, we don't know how to do anything without these two tools. This is all that we know to do: we are constantly evaluating, comparing and trying to meet expectations. Comparing yourself and fearing that you will not meet expectations is the major source of stress in your life. In jobs where the expectations are very high, and you have to constantly push yourself by comparison, you put a lot of stress on yourself and your loved ones.

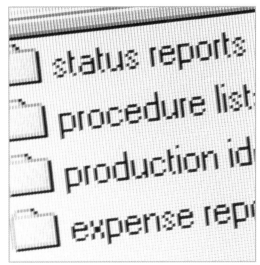
More expectations from your job could be a source of stress.

Expectations also play a very demanding role in relationships. Most of our relationships fail because we don't meet the other person's expectations, whether they are our mother's, father's, son's, wife's, boyfriend's, employ-ee's, employer's etc. Expectations can change without giving any notice to the other, and through comparison, we are expected to fulfill them. It is only because of love that we make it through relationships; if their success were left only to expectations, we all would be living alone.

A lot of times, we live our lives through others—this is especially true between parents and children. In many cases, whatever inadequacy (unfulfilled expectation) the parents feel tends to be projected onto their children. This is obviously not fair to the children because they are being put under stress at a young age and it will impact them and others for the rest of their lives. We see this behavior in our homes, on soccer fields, at baseball games and any other place where there is an expectation to be the best. Constant comparison with others takes all the focus away from the kids as individuals, which can lead to low self-esteem, insecurity and the constant fear of not being able to perform. If you don't spend your time comparing your child's performance with the others, your energy will naturally go into discovering and nurturing the talents your child already has.

Expectations and comparisons are not unique to human beings. All other species exhibit these phenomenon in one form or another. Usually an alpha male or female gives cues to the others through body language, sounds, body odor and many other mysterious ways. Expectations are defined and members of the pack need to understand and follow those by using comparisons. When one doesn't, punishments and fights try to teach what is expected.

An example of unchecked industrial pollution.

expectations and comparisons have caused an imbalance between economic development and our environment, especially in China and the United States. Since the early 1980s, China has decentralized and privatized their economic system. As a result, their gross domestic product has grown an astounding 8% year over year. However, this was achieved at the cost of polluting the environment. Now China is facing its biggest challenges in the form of pollution and major respiratory illnesses in its citizens, not to mention its contribution to global warming. China's expectation is to be as advanced as a modern western country, and its constant comparison to the United States or Western Europe has led to this imbalance. Due to our obsession with our expectations, we only look at things that favor them, which misleads us in our judgment.

Macro Impact

What we have done to ourselves, we have unconsciously done to our environment. Our

The United States has created an imbalance by trading its health and well-being for economic supremacy. The fast-paced life with high expectations has increased the speed at which people can function, causing many to lose touch with their bodies. Americans are experiencing the highest levels of obesity in the world for both adults and teenagers. Estimates and statistics show that for the first time the diseases and deaths caused by obesity are going to be higher than those caused by cigarette smoke. The health care cost in America is the highest in the world, which puts a financial strain on the health care providers and businesses. Even after spending so much money on health care there is no significant improvement in the quality of life.

Problems with Expectations and Comparisons

The problem is that they are strictly functions of your mind and hence based on calculations. However, a human being has many more functions: love, compassion and above all consciousness. Expectations and comparisons are required when you want to drive your car, ride your bicycle or write a computer program, but they are disasters when you want to have a relationship. For example, when you drive in most developed countries where there are proper roads and highways, there is a line on each side. You are expected to keep your car or bicycle in between the two lines and you use comparison to do it.

Relationships require much more complex processing of information that may have nothing to do with expectations and comparisons. In a relationship between mother and a small child, what expectations can a small child fulfill? Their love is tremendous because there are no expectations between them. With no expectations, all of their energies flow into unconditional love. It is this subtle bond that is going to last throughout their lifetime. All their lives, the mother and child will try to recreate this bond.

Are Expectations and Comparisons Natural?

In existence, there are neither expectations nor comparisons. What do you think nature (existence) is expecting from you? It has provided an abundant supply of all the life-giving energies—earth, water, air. If these things were not here, we wouldn't be here. What do we give existence in return? Nothing! We live as if existence owes us something. Nature does not compare at all because it doesn't create duplicates. Have you ever seen two identical people, flowers or animals? We are all made unique in who we are. Existence does not create clones. Cloning is a human idea. Nature is creative—which means that whatever is happening, is happening for the first time.

Expectations and comparisons are inefficient because they don't follow nature; this becomes very clear when nobody can clearly define what is expected—for example, relaxation. Can you say, "I expect to be relaxed"? It sounds comical. You cannot create an expectation out of relaxation and therefore cannot use comparison to achieve it. It would drive you insane. Say you want to relax and

you have heard that if you sit down and listen to music, you will be relaxed. You find a quiet place to sit down, close your eyes and listen to the music. In a few minutes, you experience that you are relaxing and that you are breathing deeply. However, a thought comes into your consciousness and keeps you occupied for a few seconds—and then it disappears. Once again you are back to relaxation and deep breathing. After a few seconds, another disturbing thought enters your consciousness. If you were expecting relaxation to happen by sitting down quietly, then your comparison says, "It is not happening." You will either get upset or give up. Your expectation of it will keep it at bay. You may approach your quiet times in a relaxed way, but it is not total relaxation.

You can apply the same thinking to love, sleep, meditation and other areas of your life. Like relaxation, love is a happening and cannot be created. When conditions are right, it blossoms like a flower. Due to expectations and comparisons, the process of love is disturbed and our relationship becomes a role-play of fulfilling each other's expectations.

When they are met, things are fine; when they are not, there is a problem. Reducing a relationship into a role-play kills its very essence. If you expect, then it ceases to be love.

Instead of forcing the other to conform to a certain role, have no expectations, and love will blossom. The other person's love will naturally flow because they are free of your control. Think about someone in your life that you care for. You will find that person doing things for you or loving you without expecting anything. Love without expectations is unconditional love.

Physiologically, sleep is an interesting phenomenon that impacts every part of our lives. It is like the immune system in your body that functions beautifully when everything in your life is going according to the laws of nature—both of them are interrelated. Neither the immune system nor sleep can be forced because they are a function of many processes—physiological, psychological and spiritual. You cannot force natural sleep—it is a happening. You cannot put expectations on it by saying that I will have a such-and-such type of sleep tonight. Comparing yesterday's sleep to the day before yesterday's sleep is not going to help either. It is a requirement of your body that only your body intelligence knows. All you can do is create an environment for sleep to happen. When you are tired and have no worries, sleep happens naturally to you—just like a baby.

The futility of expectations and comparisons cannot be seen more clearly than in meditation. Meditation is the expectation-less state. When you have no expectations of anything, then and only then do you come to your center. Meditation happens—it is your undisturbed, alert state. If someone says, "I meditate" or "I do meditation," they are talking about the act of meditation. Expectation and meditation are diametrically opposites.

Meditation has become almost impossible because we are creatures of expectations, and anything that is significant in our lives defies expectation. However, that is the only thing your mind knows how to do—hence the stress.

Creating an Environment and Not Expectation:

Our problem with expectation is the incorrect allocation of energy. We focus on our expectations and comparisons instead of creating the right environment. Our effort should be towards understanding and creating the right environment in anything we do. For example, if you like to

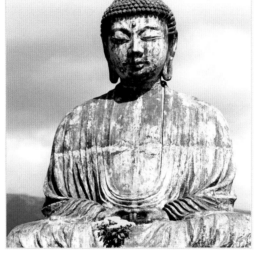

sleep well, you can burn incense, play soft music, have the room in a peaceful setting, or do some relaxing exercises before getting into bed. Once you create the right environment and you are not stressed-out mentally or physically, sleep will easily happen.

Have you seen the movie Forrest Gump? If you have not, I recommend that you do. The main character Forrest (played by Tom Hanks) had one thing that was constant throughout his life—he had no expectations! Everything simply happened to him. When he ran, he ran without expectation. When he rescued his fellow soldiers in Vietnam, he had no expectations of what would happen—he did not imagine that he could die or win a medal. Everyone who was important to him—Jenny, Lt. Dan Taylor—had expectations. Jenny had expectations to become like Joan Baez and save the world from the war. Lt. Dan Taylor wanted to die on the battlefield like his forefathers and keep the tradition alive. He was very upset to see Forrest get a medal while he was crippled and sitting in a wheelchair.

Living in expectations is not easy. Why raise the bar so high that you cannot reach it? All your life you are playing this game with yourself where you raise the bar so high and then spend your entire life jumping it and feeling like either a failure or a conqueror.

By saying, "Have no expectations," I am not saying "Don't do anything," or "Just give up." Absolutely not! I am saying, "Do everything, but don't expect anything from it." Say you have seeds of your favorite flower that you would like to plant in your garden. You get directions on how to plant the seed: you dig a hole in the ground, place the seed in the hole, cover it up with the earth and make sure it has everything to help it grow. You water the plant as required and every day come and look at the spot where you planted the seed. One day, you see a little green plant coming out of the earth. You created an environment for the plant to grow, but you did not grow the plant. If you had not created the right environment, you would never have been able to see the plant. Other things beyond your control could have happened; insects could have eaten the seed or you might have had a flood. Your whole effort of understanding and creation became a great source of transformation and joy.

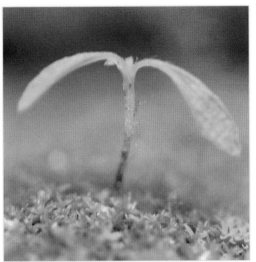

By planting the seed, you have done your part; now let existence do its part. Without expectations, you will be surprised at the many possible outcomes. Let existence surprise you with its mysteries.

What Does One Do?

No matter what you do, you can easily say that there is some element of expectation. The truth is that nature doesn't follow what you think; you have to know and follow its ways. You are not bigger than nature or existence. You are not asking for existence to fulfill your individual desires, but you want to find out things as they are and how you fit in it. It is like a puzzle. If you understand the whole picture then maybe you can see how each piece fits together. Understanding that you are a part of the whole universe and not some isolated piece is your first step.

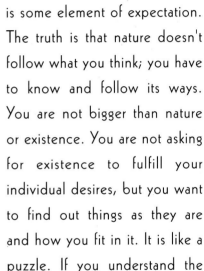

Practicing Non-Expectation

The impact of non-expectation can be seen clearly in your body by doing the following simple exercises. Once you see the difference in your body, you will be able to relate to the experience and apply it in other places. The exercises are just empty boxes; the content is the non-expectation and the non-comparison. As you pour the content, it will illuminate the container—your body. The experience will go deep into your consciousness and work its way into your relationships, work, sleep, and relaxation, eventually becoming totally you.

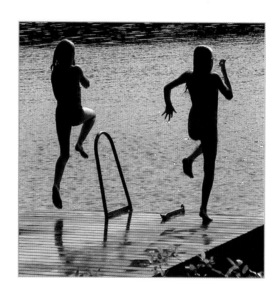

When doing the yoga stretches, at times you might feel some pain or discomfort. This is your body complaining as you try to change it. Perhaps certain muscles, tendons, ligaments or cartilages have not moved for some time. When your consciousness guides the movement, it will know exactly what to do. The consciousness will relax and dilate (open and loosen) your body and you will encounter less pain. It is like when you are trying to start an old piece of equipment. You have to do several things to get it up and running. This is exactly what you are going to encounter. Just remember—no expectations and no comparisons.

Clearing the Chatter

Keep your eyes open and sit or stand. Looking straight ahead with soft eyes, be still. Stay in this position for at least ten minutes. Don't move or look for anything; simply sit or stand without any expectation. You are doing this for no particular reason—just doing it.

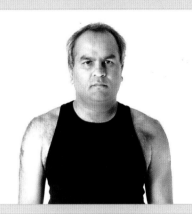

Qi-gong Rocker

Sit with your eyes closed (sit on a chair if you cannot sit on the floor). Place your palms next to your hips and bend your elbows. Slowly move your body back and forth from the lower spine. If you can imagine that you are doing this movement sitting in a swimming pool or ocean it will help.

Keep rocking your body back and forth gently without any expectations. You are not worried about the fact that you may be doing it wrong. Keep moving for the next two to three minutes.

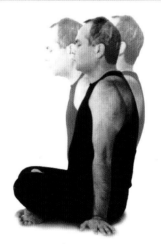

Qi-gong Head Movement

With your eyes closed and back straight, gently bring your head down until your chin touches the space between your collarbones. Then gently lift and move your head all the way back until it can go no further. Hold it there for few seconds and gently come down to the center. Then move your head all the way to the left and then to the right. Then bring your head to the center. Remember, no expectations or comparisons about these movements.

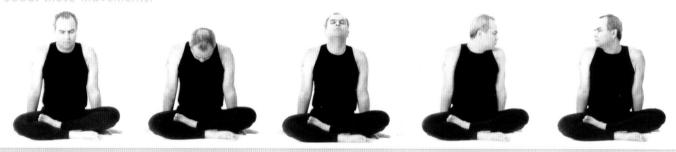

Body Energizing Qi-gong Movement

You can do this exercise either standing up or sitting down. Move your arms up and down gently without any expectations or comparisons. Move them for at least three minutes.

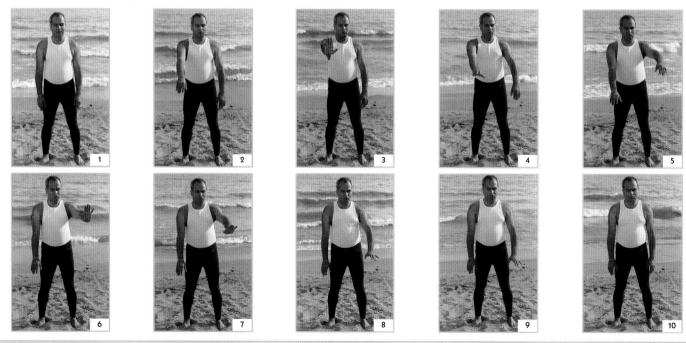

Just sit.

If you have intermittent chatter then listen to it.

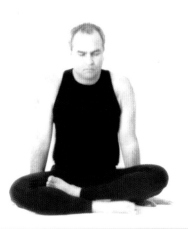

The silence that you may be feeling from these movement exercises is a direct result of your non-expectation. Your movements will become totally free because it is your expectations—of what they should do for you—that bind you. You will feel less distracted by noises around you and come into a state of deep oneness that was hard to imagine before. You have come to a state of total relaxation—in the present.

Each of the next four chapters will end with a series of exercises which will give you a taste of silence and oneness that is absolutely necessary for you to experience the state of consciousness.

When in the Real World

The information you have learned in this chapter is useful only if you can successfully apply it while you are in the real world or the "marketplace." You are a husband, a wife, a son, a daughter, a manager, a father, a mother, an employee and much more. It is hard to keep all of these roles intact and be able to do everything right. To add another level of difficulty, you may have stress from your jobs, your health, economy, religion and government policies.

At the end of each chapter, you will find out how to practically apply the information that you have received. During the day, while you are fulfilling your roles, you might feel imbalanced. In those moments, step back, evaluate your situation and see how you can apply the information you have learned. What is your expectation of the situation? Who are you comparing yourself to? As you become aware of your expectations, you will start to catch yourself before they take hold of you. This awareness will bring you to the present moment and

the entire stress process will pass without causing any disruption. Over a period of two to three months, this process will become your second nature.

On a daily basis, you are going to encounter problems with meeting and fulfilling expectations and then constantly comparing yourself to satisfy them. When you find yourself in distress, step back and look at the expectations that are imposed both by yourself and others. If these expectations cannot be met then be honest and let everyone know what you can do and what you cannot. By doing this, you will not beat up yourself or others up for no reason.

Everything that you do will originate from some expectation. You will have the most difficulty when you have expectations about things that are beyond your control. Evaluate your situation, and try not to put yourself in such positions. When you love someone, have no expectations. That may sound very counterintuitive, but it is the only thing that will work. We put more expectations on the people we love most and hence have more problems with them—we translate love into high expectations. Expectation is a poison that will ruin anything significant in your life.

Spend more time creating an environment where things will work. If you create an environment, you have done your part. However, if you try to control the outcome it will be like trying to put a bridle on a wild horse—it will be rough. In whatever you are doing, find out what would constitute the right environment, then relax and watch what happens. Things will become easy and clear.

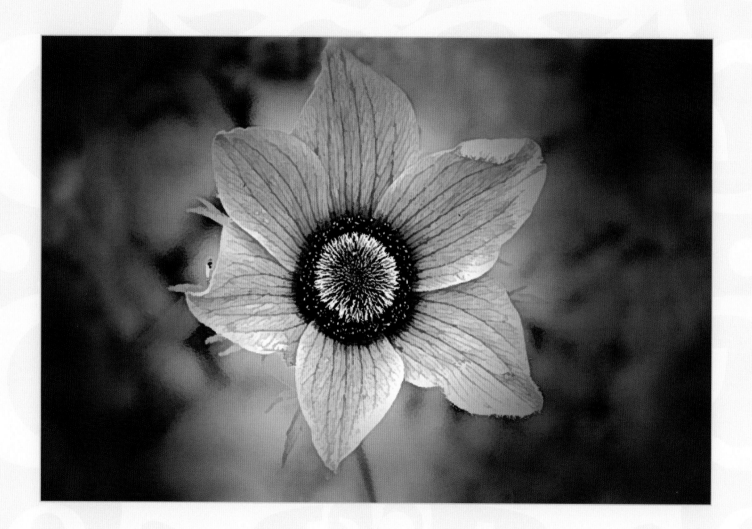

तदा सर्व आवरण मल अपेतस्य ज्ञानस्य आनन्त्यात् ज्ञेयं अल्पम्

Tada sarva aavarana mala apetasya jnaanasya aanantyaat jneyam alpam.

The sutra says, "When the veils of impurities are removed,
the highest, pure infinite knowledge of consciousness is attained;
the things that are known in it become trivial."

Patanjali, Kevalya Pada, IV-3

To clarify the essence of this sutra, imagine you are in a dark room. Naturally you will have fear and concern because you don't know what lies in front of you. You will have to spend a lot of time analyzing each move or each thing you stumble across to make sure you are safe. Now imagine that you find a switch that turns on the light in the room; all of a sudden analyses and fear will not clutter your consciousness. Finding the light switch and turning it on is comparable to lifting the veils or removing the impurities from your consciousness. Once the veils are removed your consciousness will shine like the light, not fixating on things, only observing and reflecting. You can see clearly and move safely.

One thing we all experience is chatter. The chatter of thoughts that disturbs the consciousness is what I call "The Mind." When chatter is overwhelming, you have totally become a mind, but when there is no chatter, you have become the consciousness. When you experience chatter, your body becomes stiff and dehydrated, whereas when you have no chatter, your body is loose, relaxed and hydrated. The mind is the reason for the disturbance between the body and consciousness. It is like the static noise in the reception of a radio—radio being the body, and a perfect reception being the consciousness.

The mind is an unbiased mechanism of storing information in your memory. If while collecting and storing information your consciousness was not present, then what you are storing is not going to be much help. If while collecting information you are totally conscious, then what is collected is not only stored correctly, it is also going to help several other processes in your being.

Say you are cleaning a table in your house. If there is enough light, and you can see the table with dirt and dust on it, you can do a good job. Once the table is clean, you are done and you move on to other things. However, if there is no light and you cannot see anything, then if you get all the dirt or dust off of it, it will be a miracle. Also, if you get all the dirt and dust off, how are you going to know that your work is completed? This is a problem that we all face in life. We don't know when to stop. Without the light of consciousness going through you, everything that you do will result in unfulfilling events. All types of obsessive/compulsive behavior are basically doing things in darkness where you are unable to tell when to stop.

I have never met a person who is not aware of their chatter. Chatter is the cause of stress. By constantly alerting your immune system and wearing it out, it reduces your body's ability to fight any disease, which is why it can be called the number-one killer in the world. Ironically, we have solutions to fight heart disease or cancer, but there is no cure for stress. Stress can happen on the spur of the moment and can have lasting effects on the body. Sometimes it might take years of therapy to absolve one stress memory from your life. Stress seems to be a vast phenomenon that no one medicine or therapy can completely cure.

Stress causes a runaway phenomenon of inflammation in the body. A study published in The Journal of Psychosomatic Research by Dr. P.H. Black shows that "The inflammatory events caused by stress may account for approximately 40% of atherosclerotic patients with no other known risk factors." Inflammation is a defense response caused by tissue damage or injury and characterized by redness, heat, swelling, and pain. Imagine while jogging, you fall and get cuts and bruises. These cuts and bruises become avenues for germs and bacteria to come into your body and attack it. Your body responds to this attack by localizing and eradicating the irritant and repairing the surrounding tissue. Inflammation is a necessary process of your immune system that helps you survive. The problem

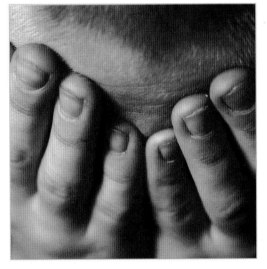

happens when the inflammation does not stop. Today experts are finding a strong relationship between all major diseases and inflammation in the body. A lot of studies are showing that a high level of inflammation in the body is a significant predictor of heart attack, stroke, diabetes, and Alzheimer's. Most research today is focused on defining and evaluating this relationship in greater detail to develop common solutions.

In stress, you get completely stiff and dehydrated, and your face and other parts of your body get very hot. This heat is caused by unprocessed emotions that do not find an outlet, which leads to inflammation in your body. The same thoughts (mind-chatter) keep on fueling those emotions over and over creating fear, anxiety, depression and many more psychological ailments. The problem is that when a particular chatter becomes a part of your consciousness, it gets an unlimited supply of energy to fulfill itself.

The important part is how we deal with mind-chatter (stress). Our usual choices are alcohol, food, sex, and drugs (both legal and illegal). We want to numb the chatter to get a break from it. Depleted and over-whelmed, your body is not capable of taking any more stress. However, because the causes are not clearly identified the solutions are only short-term, keeping the internal turmoil alive. Medically, we manage the symptoms by using psychotropic drugs, which now are given even to preschoolers. Unfortunately, even the doctors who are writing prescriptions for these drugs are divided on their long-term effectiveness. Warning labels such as: "can cause harm to the liver," or "may become prone to

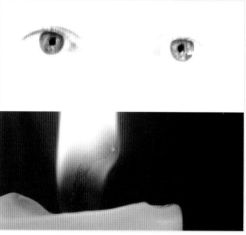

The Seeing Principle and The Light Principle

suicide," or "may lose vitality and sexual desire," are not uncommon on our medications. Unless we identify, understand and deal with the cause of mind-chatter, it is simply not going to disappear. The solution is to understand, find, and remedy the cause of chatter, thus bringing you to a state of consciousness.

The Nature of Thoughts

To see anything, we need to have two things: light and eyes. If you want to see your palm, you need to have enough light and, of course, your eyes to see it. For example, with no lights and total darkness you will not able to see your palm, or if there is light, but you are blindfolded, once again, you will not be able to see.

When you close your eyes, you see nothing but darkness. An image or a thought that comes into your head has to have two things:

- It has to be illuminated—or how else can you see it in the darkness?

- You have some type of internal seeing mechanism. Without a seeing mechanism, how would you see the thought or know that you had a thought?

Close your eyes and think about your kitchen. You will get colorful, detailed images of furniture or other things unique to your kitchen that are clearly illuminated. At the moment, these images are the only things that you will see. So you understand that your thoughts do have illumination and something within you does see these thoughts (images).

These two points are important in understanding your chatter. When you have a thought, at any given time it is the only thing that is illuminated in your head. Your internal eyes can only see what is illuminated, so they see the thought or the image against the black background. Naturally, your internal eyes start to develop a very intense alertness to the illumination (thoughts). Once this relationship matures, they get fixated on the illumination and they move with the same intensity and frequency as the thought. This fixation is the cause of chatter.

How Does Fixation Impact Us?
Say you go to see a movie in a dark theater. Since the only things you can see in the theater are the images, you get involved (fixated) with them and

forget yourself. When you forget who you are, you identify with the images. You become a part of the story (images)—crying with it, laughing with it or even talking to it. You realize you are watching a movie when someone makes you aware of it, or when the movie is over and the lights are turned on.

The same principle applies to your thoughts. Since they are the only illuminated things in your head, you easily identify with them. Once you identify with your thoughts, you cry with them, you laugh with them and often talk to them. Now, wherever the images move, your inner eyes move with them. This fixation completely drains your energy. Once fixated, you never question the thoughts that come to you and then you gamble all your energy on them.

There are some interesting similarities between the movie and the chatter in your head:

• When you are watching a movie or having a thought, you have every option to get out. You can always choose not watch the movie or entertain a thought.

• While you are watching a movie or having a thought, you are only living it temporarily. It will have a permanent effect only if it keeps replaying in your consciousness.

• While you are watching the movie or having a thought, you do not actually take part in it. It is because you identify with the characters that you feel like you are a part of them.

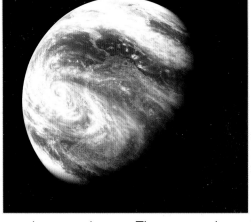

• Like the movie, thoughts happen after the fact and not in real time. Illuminated thoughts are past experiences or the projected future. In either case, you are unconscious of the present—only becoming conscious once the internal fixation is removed.

This fixation with thoughts can continue as dreams all through the night. When you have a dream, you are completely fixated with the images to the extent that it is hard for you to break away. In dreams, your fixation and identification with

thoughts is more intense. If you are active and see images all night, your body will not rest and you will be tired the next day. Once your sleep is disturbed, you will have physical and psychological problems.

What are Thoughts?

Imagine you are sitting in a dark room with a regular 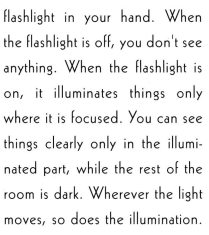 flashlight in your hand. When the flashlight is off, you don't see anything. When the flashlight is on, it illuminates things only where it is focused. You can see things clearly only in the illuminated part, while the rest of the room is dark. Wherever the light moves, so does the illumination.

The same thing happens when you close your eyes—you see nothing but darkness. Information gathered from experiences is stored as memory all over your body, but it is hidden in the dark like the room. Now imagine an internal flashlight that moves within your body and illuminates these memory banks. Whatever the flashlight illuminates, only that part of the body (memory) is revealed. Thoughts are nothing but illuminated memory spaces, while the flashlight is your intermittent level of conscious energy in your body.

What is Attention Deficit?

Imagine moving a flashlight swiftly from one side to another in a dark room. You may see things for a moment, but you will not be able to point them out clearly. This is because the movement of the flashlight was faster than what you can see and remember. The same thing happens when the internal flashlight moves at a speed that is higher than you can comprehend. You have information, but you have no comprehension. Without comprehension, the information becomes a source of stress and does not help you in taking the next step. So the act happens, but nothing is gained from it—this is lack of focus. Without focus, you will have a difficult time doing anything—you will be stressed.

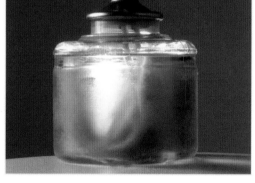

OK! We Know the Problem, but What is the Solution?

The solution is simple if you become conscious of how the energy flows through your body. Think of this energy flow as a stream that moves through your body. It starts from the soles of your feet and moves up through the top of your head. You know very well that if you place a big rock in the middle of a stream, it will alter the course of the water. Right where the water hits the rock, there will be the sound of water hitting the rock and turbulence depending on the speed of the water. Your thoughts are like the rock in the stream of your consciousness and they create the turbulence in it.

Simple Qi-gong exercises will help you experience the energy flow in your body. A proper understanding of what the exercises are trying to accomplish is critical for you to have a clear experience. Think of your body as an oil lamp. An oil lamp has three components:

a) The wick is like your head—more specifically, the center of your brain—hypothalamus, pineal and pituitary glands.

b) The container is like your body itself.

c) The fuel is like the energy that is created and flows throughout your body due to a harmonious working of all the parts.

Ideally, you want the fuel to rise through the wick and come to the top. In the same way, when doing the exercises, you want to encourage the energy to rise through the body and come to the center of the brain (hypothalamus, pituitary and pineal glands). Once this region is soaked with energy you will find that you are a part of this entire universe and you could not bring in a thought if you tried.

Step 1: Alertness Technique

Stand with your feet apart (shoulder width) keeping your head straight and eyes open. Try to be extremely still. Don't focus on anything in particular; just have a soft gaze. Relax your whole body especially your feet, legs and stomach. All exercises are to be done in bare feet whenever possible. Stand in this position for 10 to 12 minutes. Don't expect to see anything in particular—just stand, look straight ahead and relax.

Think of the energy moving through your body as airflow or cross-ventilation in your house. When the windows are open and breeze flows through your house without any blocks, it will keep it cool and fresh. In the same way, think of a window in the soles of your feet and another window in the top of your head. Let the energy flow through and you will feel freshness and vitality.

A Path of Energy Flows Through Your Body

When you are standing in an upright position and in a totally relaxed state, you will notice that points in

Hypothalamus

Pituitary Gland

Pineal Gland

Managing Expectations and Comparisons

the soles of your feet (Yongquan cavity or the bubbling wells) will get energized and you will feel a sense of connection with the earth. Similarly, there are points on your palms (Laogong cavity) from which you will feel the connection. (For more details see chapter 10.)

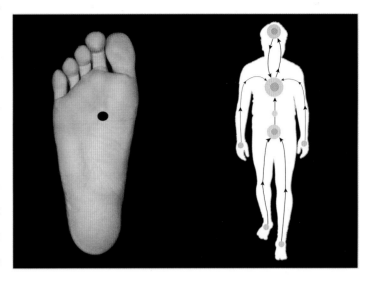

Once you are totally relaxed, the energy will automatically flow from the soles of your feet (Yongquan) through the top of your head (Gu Shen) like a hollow tube. The oil lamp example will help you move the energy from the soles to the center of your brain, the hypothalamus (Xuan Guan). Once the energy moves and soaks the hypothalamus, it will remain there. In this state, you will experience the deepest silence because now information is coming into the brain without any expectations or comparisons clouding what you are seeing, hearing, touching, smelling and tasting. The silence will be so strong that it will feel like someone has squeezed all the chatter out of you. This process is the most advanced form of Qi-gong training called Kai Qio.

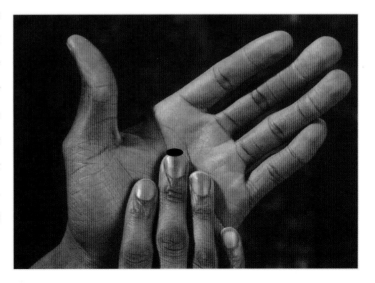

Step 2: Relaxation Exercises:

These five exercises will help you experience the space of oneness in and around you. Once you have this experience, you can use any exercise from Chapter 10. When you have learned to balance, you will know how to slip into the state of deep relaxation.

Some tips:

1) Move into all of the exercises like they are happening to you; you are not the doer - no expectations.

2) Once you have familiarized yourself with the exercises, then keep your eyes closed.

3) Feel like you are in water for all of the exercises and imagine that your body is like a grain of salt dissolving into the water. When your body (matter) is dissolved into energy (water or consciousness) it can flow from one form to the next with ease and total focus.

4) Feel all of the stretches and movements originating from the lowest part of the spine.

5) Breathe naturally and never hold your breath.

You will find that certain core exercises are repeated from one chapter to the next. The repetition will do two things: make you familiar with the core exercises, and help you learn how to come into a state of total relaxation with ease. For you to be able to come to your spiritual self, how you do the exercises is important. If you do the slow-moving Qi-gong exercises in the way described above, you will find strength and energy beyond your wildest dreams. You will be able to go to the source of energy directly. This will give you a new perspective about who you are, and at that point in your inner stillness, you will be able to make better decisions for yourself.

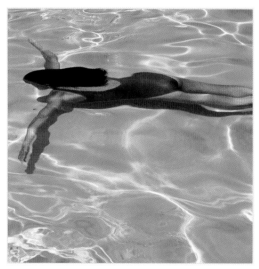

Swimming in Consciousness.

Wear loose clothing and use a yoga mat. Yoga mats are available at many health and department stores. If you have difficulty sitting on the floor you can use a simple chair without side arms. Remember, while doing the exercises—have no expectations or comparisons—either of yourself or others. For best results, these 20-minute exercises should be done twice a day for at least 21 to 30 days.

Three Main Energy Centers in the Body

When your mind totally relaxes, all the energy used by the brain is released. This energy then moves to your heart and ultimately to the third dan-tian, or energy plexus (what the Japanese call the "hara"). In the Eastern system of human understanding, the third dan-tian is your brain center. When your energy moves into the third dan-tian you will be able to see, listen to and understand things far more clearly. Imbalances in the body occur where the energy is blocked—99% of the time it is in the head, because we use our mind for nearly everything. Very rarely does our energy come to the second or third dan-tian. The standing technique and certain Qi-gong and yoga exercises correct this imbalance.

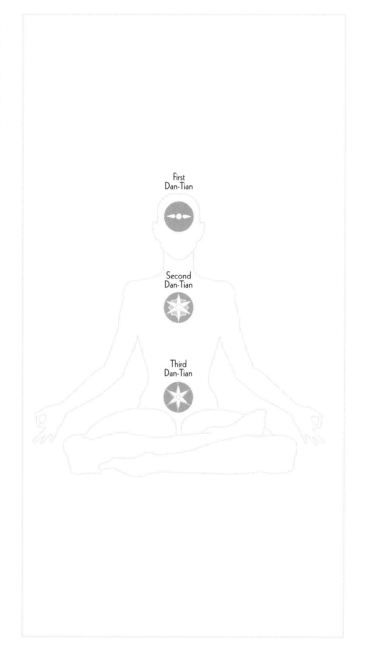

First
Dan-Tian

Second
Dan-Tian

Third
Dan-Tian

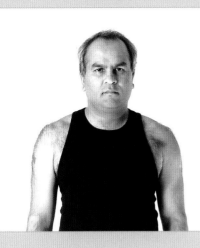

Clearing the Chatter

Keep your eyes open and sit or stand. Looking straight ahead with soft eyes, be still. Stay in this position for at least ten minutes. Don't move or look for anything; simply sit or stand without any expectation. You are doing this for no particular reason—just doing it.

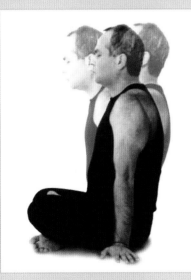

Qi-gong Rocker

Sit with your eyes closed (sit on a chair if you cannot sit on the floor). Place your palms next to your hips and bend your elbows. Slowly move your body back and forth from the lower spine. If you can imagine that you are doing this movement sitting in a swimming pool or ocean it will help.

Keep rocking your body back and forth gently without any expectations. You are not worried about the fact that you may be doing it wrong.
Keep moving for the next two to three minutes.

Managing Expectations and Comparisons

Qi-gong Head Movement

With your eyes closed and back straight, gently bring your head down until your chin touches the space between your collarbones. Then gently lift and move your head all the way back until it can go no further. Hold it there for few seconds and gently come down to the center. Then move your head all the way to the left and then to the right. Then bring your head to the center. Remember no expectations or comparisons about these movements.

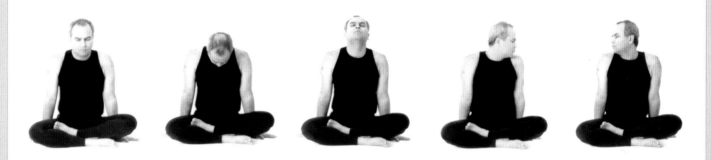

Janu Sirsasan (Head on Knees)

Without breaking the silence, bring your left foot out and your right foot next to your left thigh. Slowly start to move your chin towards your left knee while keeping your knee straight. Feel like you are pouring into this form. Stay in this position for at least two to three minutes. As always, with any stretch, you are ready to move to the next only when you have become relaxed in the form.

Change sides and bring your left foot next to your right thigh, keeping your right knee straight. Gently lower your chin towards your right knee. No expectations and no comparisons to the other side. Feel the stretch coming from the lowest part of the spine. Stay in this form until you have become totally relaxed.

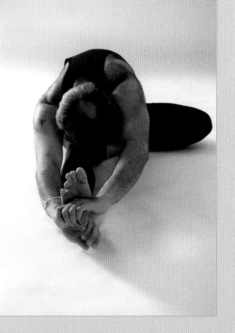

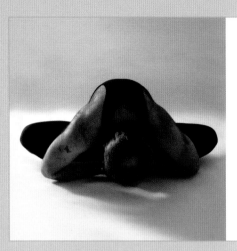

Baddha Konasana (Restraint Angle Stretch)

Bring both soles of your feet next to each other. If this feels too tight then bring your left foot over your right leg. Do the best you can, even if this feels tight as well. Bring your head forward, stretching from the lowest part of the spine. Stay in this form until you are totally relaxed.

This stretch may be hard to do if you are a beginner.

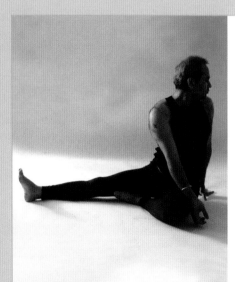

Sitting Lower Spine Twist

Softly and easily, place your left foot on top of your right thigh. Place your left arm behind your spine and your right palm over your left knee. Feel the stretch in the back of your body and lower spine. Keep your eyes closed and stay in the stretch until totally relaxed.

No expectations or comparisons.

Change sides, repeat the exercise and stay in the form for three to four minutes. Once you are able to stretch fully, it will be very effective in letting the energy flow from the base of your spine to your head.

Becoming-One Qi-gong Movement

Qi-gong is the only thing that will fully show you the power of no-expectation. Let your arms rise up to the side without your doing. Keep moving your arms up and down for next three to five minutes. Slowly and gently.

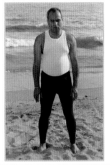 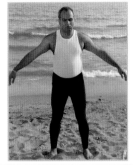 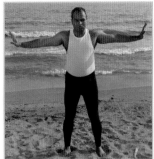 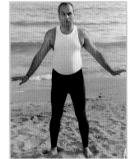 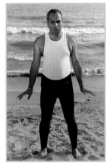

Body Energizing Qi-gong Movement

Move your arms up and down gently without any expectations or comparisons. With each move of your arms, feel the relaxation and let the energy rise into the center of the brain. Move them for at least three minutes.

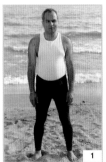 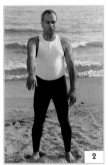 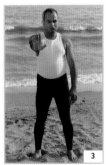 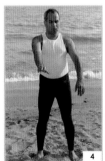 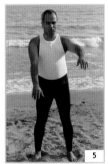

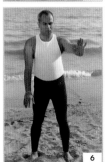 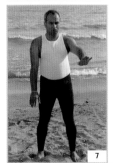 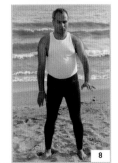 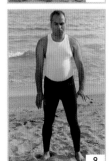 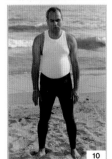

Body Balancing Qi-gong Movement

Bring both of your palms facing upwards below your navel. Gently let your palms rise up like someone is lifting them up for you. When your palms pass your heart center turn them around and let the palms start to flow downwards until they cross over the navel. Repeat the movement for two to three minutes gently.

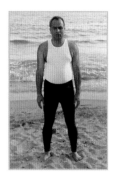 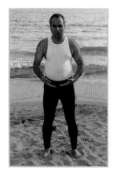 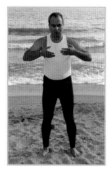 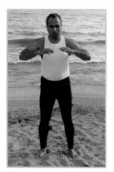 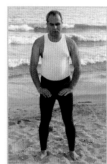 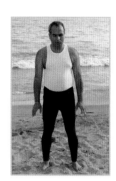

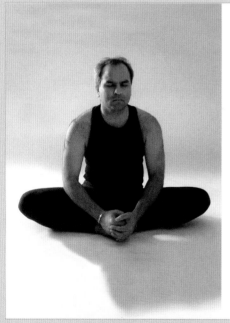

Ah Ha Asana (Sukha Asana, Blissful Posture)

If you are completely relaxed by now, you may want to take a break and just experience the silence.

Sit in silence and keep your eyes closed for as long as you like. You will not be able to tell where you begin and where you end. By doing these exercises every day you will familiarize yourself with the silent space-making it your default state. Once you feel comfortable, you may want to add more exercises from Chapter 10 that will help you go further into your body and consciousness.

What Happens When the Energy Flows?

The first exercise, where you stand with your feet apart and gaze, is a simple yet very powerful technique for unidentifying with internal chatter. It is a meditation because it breaks the fixation between the thought and the internal-eye movement. Even one experience with this technique will go a long way in reducing chatter. Our eyes and mind are trained to focus on objects and not the space between the objects. This is the cause of constant chatter, because we never get a break in between thoughts. This technique will help you become aware of the space in between thoughts.

Doing the slow-moving Qi-gong exercises and remembering the oil lamp example will help you understand and feel your essence and vitality. In anything that happens to you, your brain collects and processes the information at different locations. Then it sends the information to its center—the hypothalamus. The hypothalamus then signals its messengers, the pituitary and

Hormone Production and the Major Physiologic Effect of the Pituitary Gland

	Hormone	Major Target Organ(s)	Major Physiologic Effects
Anterior (Front) Pituitary	Growth hormone	Liver, adipose tissue	Promotes growth (indirectly), controls of protein, lipid and carbohydrate metabolism
	Thyroid-stimulating hormone	Thyroid gland	Stimulates secretion of thyroid hormones
	Adrenocorticotropic hormone	Adrenal gland (cortex)	Stimulates secretion of glucocorticoids
	Prolactin	Mammary gland	Milk production
	Luteinizing hormone	Ovaries and testes	Controls reproductive function
	Follicle-stimulating hormone	Ovaries and testes	Controls reproductive function
Posterior (Back) Pituitary	Antidiuretic hormone	Kidney	Conserves body water
	Oxytocin	Ovaries and testes	Stimulates milk secretion and uterine contractions

pineal glands, which release specific types of hormones informing other glands and parts of your body what needs to be done. One example would be prolactin, a hormone produced by the anterior (front) pituitary gland in both men and women. It is known as a gonadotrophic hormone because it affects the gonads (testes and ovaries). It also has an effect on other organs in the body. In males, prolactin influences the production of testosterone and effects sperm production. If prolactin secretion is increased, testosterone levels drop and sperm production is reduced or absent, resulting in male infertility. The table shows some of the hormones that are produced and released by the pituitary gland.

If you imagine inserting your finger between your eyebrows, going all the way to the center of your brain, you will "touch" your pineal gland. In the last decade, the pineal gland has gotten a lot of attention because it produces melatonin, a very important hormone. It is the one that regulates sleep, rejuvenates the immune system and reverses the aging process. Melatonin has shown unprecedented results in lab experiments with mice. A lot of research is currently being done on this mysterious pea-sized gland's effect on other critical functions of our body. For an in-depth account of the relationship between the pineal gland, melatonin and the body, please read "The Melatonin Miracle" by Drs. Pierpaoli and Regelson.

Through experiments, scientist today are finding out that our body's ability to fight diseases slows down as we age because of the following factors:

1) Over the years, the communication between the hypothalamus, pituitary and adrenal glands is stressed and not what it used to be when you were younger.

2) There is no rest for these glands when they are working day and night to keep the body functioning. Fatigued, they become unable to produce critical hormones at the required levels.

3) The glands themselves can become diseased.

The key here is rest. When you do the exercises and let the energy come up to the center of the brain, you will find that for the first time in your life you have tasted rest. The critical organs in your brain are replenished. They get a long-overdue break. You will feel a tremendous sense of physiological relaxation—physiological in the sense that you are not telling yourself to relax, but your body is in a deep state of relaxation. In the East, they call this state "Samadhi," where you are totally alert yet totally relaxed. You will find that your breath will become extremely deep and slow and may even stop intermittantly. Don't panic! This is a good indication that your mind is inactive. Not one thought will be able to pass through your head even if you wanted. It is a complete stoppage of all activity. Once you taste this space of stillness, you recognize that you have found what you have been looking for all along. Now you will not need sex, drugs, food, money, power, ego, prestige or other things. Your search will be over, and you will find contentment under your feet.

Is Silence Boring?

One question often raised is: Wouldn't it be boring to have no thoughts? Or, without thoughts, how can you be spontaneous?

When you are in a state where you have no chatter, it does not mean that you will cease to do things. On the contrary, you will be doing things more efficiently—without any disturbance. You will not have to read a paragraph five times before you get it. You will continue your life just the way it was, but there will be a tremendous internal qualitative difference because you are not going back and forth with your thoughts. When you have chatter, it is like trying to walk with one leg and crutches. When you have no chatter, you have both legs to walk.

With chatter, you cannot be truly spontaneous. We confuse spontaneity with impulsiveness. To be spontaneous, you need to be totally aware, open and not stuck in some crisis. Being spontaneous is a highly creative event because you respond to what is in front of you and totally connect to whatever you're doing. Impulsiveness, on the other hand, is a desperate effort to break away from the rut of your mind. You are connected to your thoughts. You may do things that you will regret when you are impulsive, but that is not the case when you are spontaneous.

A chattering mind is like driving in the night without headlights. It may feel more thrilling and exciting, but it keeps you tense and you don't learn or enjoy anything. Living on the edge all the time and going from one mistake to another makes you feel occupied, but it is a very ineffective system. Imagine working in a poorly-lit room all the time. You will have little idea of what is clearly happening and you will lose the capacity to see. This is what happens with us. Working in darkness and disturbance, we lose clear vision and living without clarity feels normal. You can only do things that you know or have experienced. It is hard for you to imagine or function without any chatter. That is the only normal thing you know.

Modern psychologists try to analyze your chatter and make sense of it. Unfortunately, the chatter is the revelation of memory space by the movement of the light principle in your being, and that movement is not in your hands. You cannot predict what your next thought is going to be. Your inward eyes are fixated on the internally-illuminated thoughts that are the roots of your problems. So far, we have not made much progress. On the contrary, the fixation has become deeper. All the violence and destruction that we see doesn't seem to bother us anymore. Our real lives have become like a movie where we are identified with the characters and really cannot do much about anything. We keep on watching and do nothing—our eyes are open, but there is little comprehension.

When in the Real World

There are going to be days when the chatter will be overwhelming and draining. These will reduce if you have a daily practice regiment. I have put together a DVD "Introduction to Consciousness" including the exercises, or you can check www.Athmo.com for new material. If you use the above exercises like a pill, doing them only when you have a problem, they will not be very effective. The meditative exercises are like brakes for your mind. While driving, when you want to slow down your car, you apply the brakes way before you get close to the car that is in front of you. If you apply brakes only when you are about to hit another car, the brakes will be ineffective.

Create a regiment for yourself and try not to miss it. At work or any other place where you feel you have a lot of chatter disturbing your consciousness, take a break and find a silent space. At work you can shut your office door, or go to the bathroom, or step outside the office building. You only need ten minutes to rejuvenate. Relax your whole body and do the slow-moving Qi-gong exercises one, two, six, seven, and eight. Letting the energy flow to the center of your brain (remember the oil lamp) will rejuvenate your body and bring you to your consciousness. The chatter will be completely gone and it may be hard for you to leave this space of silence. This ten-minute silent break can become a new tool in your collection to successfully bring your body and consciousness into balance.

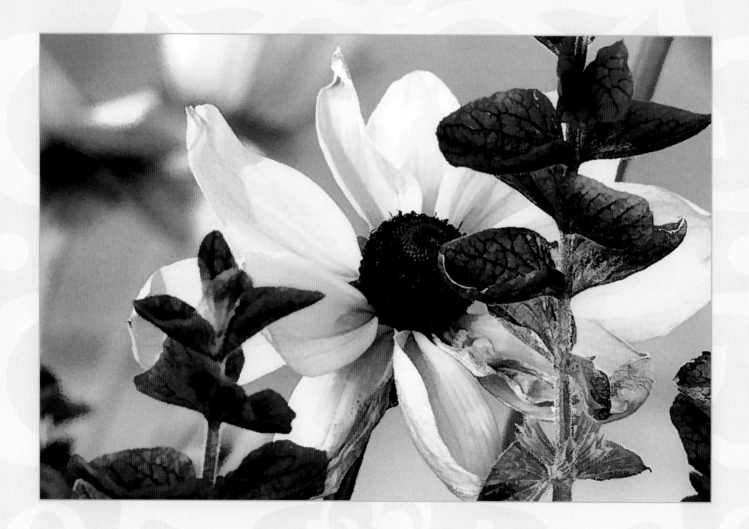

Soul receives from soul that knowledge,
therefore not by book
nor from tongue.

If knowledge of mysteries comes
after emptiness of mind,
that is illumination of heart.

Mevlana Jalal-e-Din Mevlavi Rumi

What is Virtual Reality?

A constant fixation on a particular thought makes it real in your mind and gives it a reality that only you can understand. This can have far-reaching repercussions. If a constant thought that "I am going to fail in a certain event" runs through your mind over and over, then you will have a hard time being successful in it. Even though your thought may not have any validity, it has brought about a real effect on your mind and life. Once it becomes real, the outcome of the thought is almost predictable. When chatter keeps playing in our consciousnesses, we start to act it out. Millions of lives were lost in World War II because of Hitler's virtual reality of supremacy. He thought that he and people like him were the only supreme beings and he kept on repeating this lie until he was able to program a whole nation with his virtual reality.

How Chatter Becomes Reality

Imagine that you and I are having a face-to-face conversation. We talk back and forth several times, which leads to a point of agreement or disagreement.

After we part, on your way to your next stop, a thought or image of my face comes into your mind. Before you know it, an automatic conversation will begin in your mind, which can last for a few seconds to several hours. This is what we call thinking. The emotional or feeling component of the thought will determine the duration of the automatic conversation. The entire phenomenon of automatic conversation is based on the fact that you cannot tell the difference between me and your thought of me. This is "Virtual Reality." The entire process has both components: it is virtual because it is created in your head, and real because it does happen. You respond to both of them because, to you, both of them are real, and it does not matter if I am physically in front of you or not; you will talk with the image.

The problem is that the image or thought in your head is your version of me, which is, or can be, very different from who I am. Essentially, the conversation in your head is from both sides. You are speaking with your image of me. If this were a tennis match, you would be hitting the ball from both sides of the court. Remember, the real conversation we had ended a long time ago, but once this internal conversation starts, there may be no end to it because you create your own questions through my image and then answer them. We experience this endless chatter on a daily basis. Your consciousness is constantly disturbed because you can go into a self-conversation on ten different subjects in about two minute's time. In the end, you are left tired, without the energy to directly experience anything.

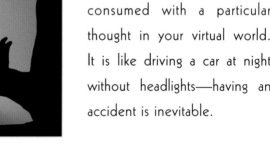

Virtual reality is the world or the movie that we create by living in the chatter. The illuminated thoughts and inner fixation discussed previously are the components that make this world or movie.

How Does it Affect Us?

When my image enters your consciousness, it can take several forms or directions with endless possibilities. If there are emotions attached to my image then you will experience even more stress. You try your hardest to answer your own questions, but somehow they never seem to end. When you are involved in an automatic act for the entire day, guess what? You will be doing the same thing at night, while you are asleep. The chatter will transform into dreams and nightmares. Once the unprocessed thoughts, emotions or feelings enter into your subconscious, their impact on your life is far-reaching.

• First, you are not conscious because your entire energy is consumed with a particular thought in your virtual world. It is like driving a car at night without headlights—having an accident is inevitable.

• Second, your tired mind is so overworked with these mental gymnastics that it is on the verge of short-circuiting every chance it gets. Much violence and mental illness in our society today is a result of this short-circuiting.

Self-Talk, Stress, Immune System and Inflammation

Impact of Images or Thoughts on Your Body

Virtual reality is created when you are engaged in self-talk with an image or thought in your head. The two components of your self-talk are the image (thought) and the response (in the form of talk that originates in your jaws). If you sit down in silence, you will find that you either will have too many thoughts coming into your head, or you will find you have a strain in your jaws because you have been speaking silently. Either way, when you are caught in a state of virtual reality, you will feel a lot of strain in your head and jaws leading you to feel stress in your face, head, neck and shoulders.

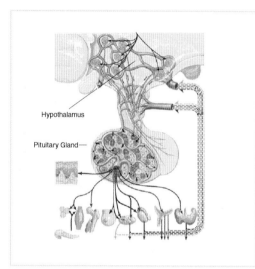

Hypothalamus

Pituitary Gland

When you have a thought illuminated in your brain, it has a far-reaching impact on the body. The information from the thought is processed in the brain and the result is sent to the hypothalamus in the center of your brain. Underneath the hypothalamus there is a master gland (the size of a pea) called the pituitary gland that works in conjunction with several other glands to keep your body in balance. The illustration shows the relationship between the pituitary gland and all the parts of the body.

The pituitary gland can be thought of as a central post office. When it receives directions from the hypothalamus to respond to a situation, it releases certain hormones that give an indication to the receptive gland to take appropriate action.

More specifically, when you are presented with a stressful situation or thought, your hypothalamus, pituitary and adrenal glands work together to bring your body into balance. The medical community identifies the trio as the HPA (hypothalamus-pituitary-adrenal) axis. First, the hypothalamus releases a compound called the corticotrophin releasing factor

(CRF). The CRF then travels to the pituitary gland, where it triggers the release of a hormone called ACTH. The ACTH is released into the bloodstream and causes the cortex of the adrenal gland to release stress hormones, particularly cortisol, a corticosteroid. Cortisol affects the availability of the fuel supply (carbohydrate, fat, and glucose metabolism), which is needed to respond to stress. However, if cortisol levels stay increased for too long then muscle breakdown, a decreased inflammatory response, and suppression of the immune (defense) system will occur.

You can imagine what happens when you have all types of thoughts entering and leaving your consciousness. A stressful thought can be followed by anger, frustration, or disgust. The pituitary gland has to produce and release hormones on the fly. To start and stop the HPA process over and over again is not healthy for your body or consciousness.

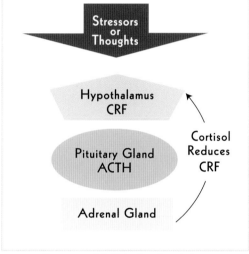

Stress and HPA feedback loop

A study by Dr. Black, "Stress, Inflammation and Cardiovascular Disease" published in the Journal of Psychosomatic Research finds, "The argument is made that humans reacting to stressors, which are not life-threatening but are "perceived" as such, mount similar stress/inflammatory responses in the arteries, which, if repetitive or chronic, may culminate in atherosclerosis." The table shown on page 53 shows all the hormones produced by the pituitary gland and their impact on different organs of the body.

The techniques explained in the previous chapter will help you to reduce thoughts and bring about a focus. As you practice the technique, you will be able to build your immune system and reduce inflammation in your body.

Impact of Self Talk on Your Body

When you are talking, several parts of the body

have to perform their respective functions—your jaws and tongue move with a certain coordination, while the diaphragm just above your stomach moves air from your lungs through the mouth. You may not be aware of it, but the same thing happens when you are having a self-conversation: your jaws move ever so slightly. When you have a long self-conversation, you will feel a certain pain and fatigue where your jaws meet.

The muscles in your mouth are used the most. For the food to be digested, it has to be properly processed in your mouth. On the sides of your mouth, as shown in the picture, you have a large parotid gland that along with smaller submaxillary and sublingual glands makes and discharges saliva. The saliva is a clear, semi-viscous liquid that helps in the digestion of food. Human saliva contains alpha-amylase, an enzyme specifically designed to break down complex carbohydrates into sugar compounds.

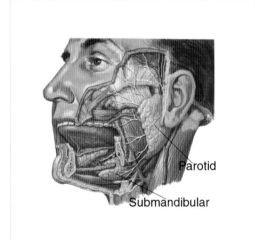

Parotid

Submandibular

When we don't chew our food properly and mix it with saliva, this process is seriously compromised. Not chewing your food properly, at least 10-15 bites, is one of the causes of obesity and food addiction.

When you have a fearful or angry response to a situation, you will notice several things. Your mouth gets dry, your face gets red and you feel heat in your whole body. You will feel that your whole body is on fire and it may even start to shake at times. When your mouth gets dry it means that there is little or no saliva. This puts a tremendous amount of stress on your salivary glands. The natural response is to lose your appetite. Both heart rate and lung activity become high, putting pressure on things that may already be at their maximum limits. As a response, your body's defense mechanism kicks in and you start to perspire to cool off. You might have a strong, natural urge to drink a glass of water to bring your body into a balance.

Interestingly enough, there is a small gland in your lower jaw underneath your tongue called the submandibular gland. Current research has shown that this gland releases certain peptides and proteins that are responsible for tissue repairs in the oral cavity, gastrointestinal tract and liver. When you have stress, your mouth—in particular the glands involved— reacts, and two things will happen:

• The whole body will become stiff which means poor or no circulation. The digestive organs, such as the stomach and intestines, will start to discharge fluids that will damage body tissue. Each time you eat, your stomach discharges hydrochloric acid to digest the food. In addition, it creates a water-based stomach lining to save the walls of the stomach. However, during stress there is no protection created, which causes major infections and diseases in the body such as acid reflux, stomach ulcers, ulcerated colitis, ulcer of the gastrointestinal tract, hemorrhoids and other inflammatory diseases.

• While the body is being damaged, the amount of enzymes and chemicals to rebuild the body are in a short supply due to the stress in the submandibular gland. This imbalance makes the situation worse and it becomes a major disease state. In many cases, this process is repeated over many days before you get medical help, so you are in unnecessary pain and discomfort. The above process can be thought of as heating an empty pan on a fire. It serves no purpose and will burn anything that is put into it.

A research study on a particular strain of rats, performed by Drs. R. D. Mathison, A. D. Befus, J.S. Davison has found that the submandibular gland performs the following critical functions in the body:

a) The submandibular gland releases peptides and proteins that facilitate tissue repair in the oral cavity, gastrointestinal tract, and more distal sites such as the liver.

b) It has been shown that salivary gland factors also modulate inflammatory responses, because they found that removal of the submandibular gland increases the responses to endotoxin.

c) From this observation they proposed that these glands contain a factor that regulates cardiovascular response to shock.

d) The data indicates that the submandibular gland participates in the regulation of your entire body (systemic homeostasis).

What Are Our Choices?

The solutions offered today by our medical profession are medication or therapy. If you are taking psychotropic medication, you know very well what I am talking about. There is a whole list of pills that work in their own unique way to help you cope with your "virtual reality." Almost all of them have side effects; in some cases they may be addiction to the medication itself.

Imagine your body as a house with a fire alarm (neurological response). Taking a pill without understanding the cause of the problem is like removing the battery or temporarily disconnecting the fire alarm as it goes off. If you remove the battery from a fire alarm, it will give the fire more time to get stronger, spreading into other areas of the house.

A Holistic Solution

All self-talk involves two things: the image or the thought in your head and your response. Your response comes from your ever-so-slight jaw movement. This tension between the image and the jaws is what needs to be relaxed or broken. Until this happens it will be impossible to go beyond chatter or any virtual reality. No amount of drugs or therapy alone will help, until the cause is identified.

The Art of Listening

We hear the constant chatter of thoughts like we hear a radio. Many times we listen to the radio because we are not comfortable being alone. To avoid this uneasy, jittery feeling we turn on the radio to replace the chatter in our head—the radio keeps us occupied. We do feel the disturbance from the chatter, but somehow or other never listen to or comprehend it. Lack of consciousness of the chatter gives it a perpetual life in our brain. Understanding this phenomenon will be key for you to become stress-free.

The solution is simple: just listen. Listen to your thoughts or any conversation that may be happening—especially where your two jaws meet. You will find that all your self-talk originates in your jaws. The best way to start would be to sit down comfortably on a chair or the floor, keep your lower jaw relaxed and listen to anything. Try not playing any music that you like because you will be active with it. Listen to anything that is naturally happening around you—birds singing, waves of the ocean, trees dancing, or your neighbor's dog barking. You are just a listener. While you are listening to things around, you will get intermittent thoughts and chatter; listen to them as well. Remember not to get involved with them—just listen. Sit and listen for at least 15 minutes. You will start to feel a sense of tremendous silence by being in this state of listening.

When you start to listen, you will find that your lower jaw is not stressed anymore—it becomes totally relaxed. When you listen intently, your whole being falls into synchronicity. You find that whenever you listen to your chatter (thoughts) it just disappears. If two people have an argument and all of a sudden one of them realizes the futility of the whole situation and just shuts up and listens, what do you think will happen to the conversation? It will end abruptly. This is an interesting phenomenon—the most stressful thing in your life disappears when you become conscious and listen to it. This is meditation. When you sit and listen you are including everything. You are not picking and choosing between what you want to listen to and what you don't. Since there are no expectations, you find that not only are you able to sit for a long time, but also you feel a sense of peace and joy. This is a taste of your consciousness.

The good thing about listening is that you can do it at any time and you will get very adept at it. Then you will be able to listen while traveling, driving your car, washing dishes, taking a walk, or just sitting. You will find that your body is naturally relaxed and has a sense of alertness that you have never felt before.

In addition, exercises can relax the tension in these muscles and glands and help you to listen. While doing the exercises keep your lower and upper jaw relaxed. How relaxed your jaw is, will become an indicator to how relaxed or tense your whole body is. You will find that the moment you relax your jaw, you have no chatter in your head.

Lotus Position (Padmasana)

Remember no expectations and no comparisons while doing the exercises. With your eyes closed, sit silently. Bring your awareness to your mouth and your lower jaw. Remember you are not concentrating on the mouth but only becoming aware of it. Keep the lower jaw totally relaxed. Stay in this space for at least ten minutes.

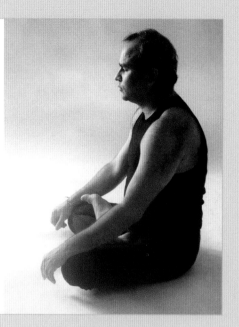

Qi-gong Rocker

Sit with your eyes closed (sit on a chair if you cannot sit on the floor). Place your palms next to your hips and bend your elbows. Slowly move your body back and forth from the lower spine. If you can imagine that you are doing this movement sitting in a swimming pool or ocean it will help.

Keep rocking your body back and forth gently without any expectations. You are not worried about the fact that you may be doing it wrong.

Keep moving for the next two to three minutes.

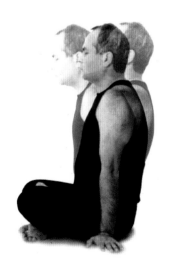

Qi-gong Head Movement

With your eyes closed and back straight, gently bring your head down until your chin touches the space between your collarbones. Then gently lift and move your head all the way back until it can go no further. Hold it there for few seconds and gently come down to the center. Then move your head all the way to the left and then to the right. Then bring your head to the center. Remember, no expectations or comparisons about these movements.

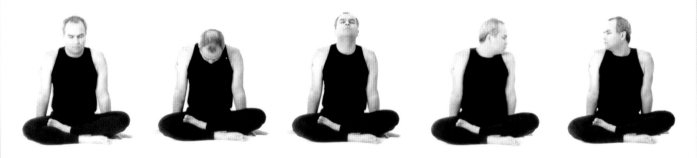

Body Balancing Qi-gong Movement

Bring both of your palms facing upwards below your navel. Gently let your palms rise up like someone is lifting them up for you. When your palms pass your heart center turn them around and let the palms start to flow downwards until it crosses over the navel. Repeat the movement for two to three minutes gently.

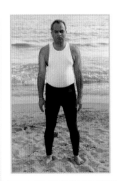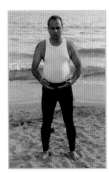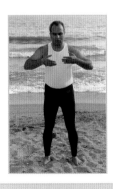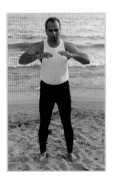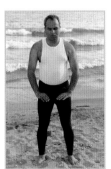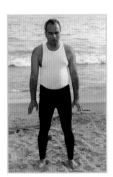

Managing Expectations and Comparisons

Heaven to Earth Qi-gong Movement

Bring your palms facing upwards to your navel and let them rise up. When your palms reach between your shoulder and face they will naturally start to flip and turn upwards. Let your palms keep rising until they cannot rise up anymore. Then let your arms move out gently with the palms facing down and start to come down towards the earth. Repeat the movement once again. When you get totally relaxed, you will feel like you are swimming in consciousness. This is exactly where you want to be.

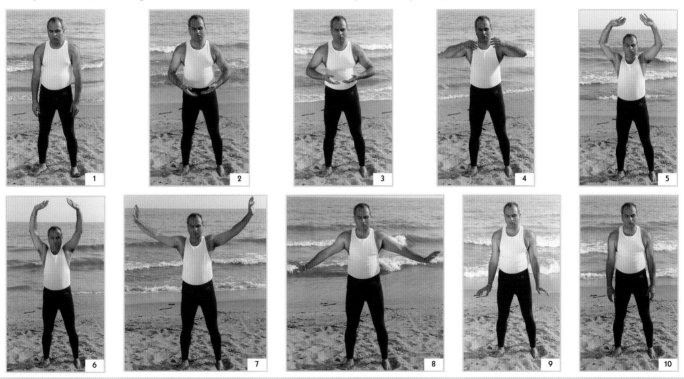

While doing these exercises you may feel a little more saliva than usual and that is OK. When you relax your mouth, it will secrete more saliva—that is exactly what should happen. Over a few days, the excess saliva should stop flowing and the mouth will start to be naturally relaxed and come into a balance. It is clear that doing the exercises alone will not help—how you do them and what you know about them is essential for their effectiveness.

In Summary

So far, you have experienced the effects of three simple things on your body: No-expectations and No-comparisons, the internal focus technique, and the listening technique. The exercises in the previous chapters helped you to experience the space of relaxation. Doing the exercises should be your number-one priority if you want to reduce chatter and have a healthy body. The exercises are easy and they will make you feel energetic.

Chapter 10, and the DVD that is designed to be used with this book, are your two main sources of exercises. In chapter 9 there are six mandatory exercises suggested to bring your body into a structural balance. All exercises should be done with no expectations and no comparisons.

Your daily routine can be anywhere from a half hour to an hour depending on your schedule. Only in very rare instances, should you miss your daily practice. Your time to exercise is time for you alone. It is one-on-one time between you and existence (nature). It is a time for you to connect with yourself and know how things are at your core. You will be able to feel any disturbances or healing in your body and mind. Make your exercise the most important thing in your life and it will become your center, keeping you grounded.

There is nothing more real in this world than virtual reality. The power of self-talk and images that engage us and determine every aspect and outcome of our life cannot be overstated. The only way a virtual reality comes to an end is when you first realize that you are having an automatic conversation with someone who is not even physically in front of you.

In any given day there will be several times when you experience virtual reality, losing consciousness of the present and who you are. When you catch yourself in these moments look at the whole situation and realize that you are not having a conversation with the real entity. When you do this about five times, you will find that it is very hard for you to slip into a state of virtual reality. It will be very easy for you to stay conscious and focused effortlessly. If you do the exercises as shown, you will not identify with thoughts and you will stay free of virtual reality.

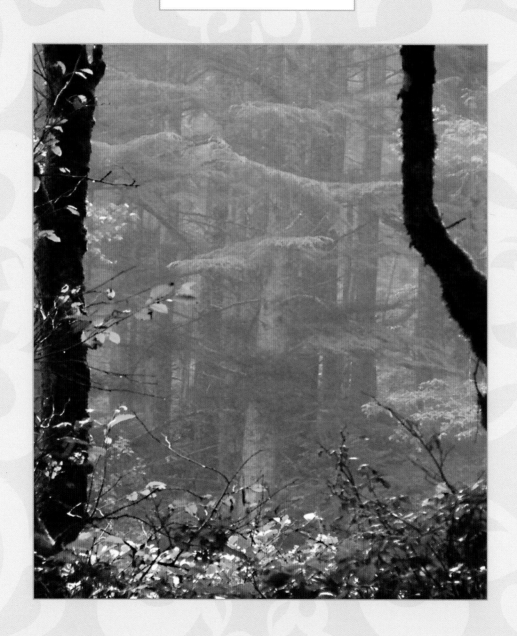

Stir the muddy water and
It will remain cloudy.

Leave it alone and
It will get clear.

Let the stream flow and
It will find its way.

Stop chasing contentment and
It will come to you.

(Chuang Tzu)

One thing common among all human beings is experience. The clarity with which we experience and remember will determine what we learn and unlearn. If the comprehension we reach through the experience is unclear, then we will have to repeat the act. This repetition is done until the experience, and through it the understanding, is clear—this is the "law of Karma." Say you are having a conversation with someone and suddenly a thought engages your consciousness. As soon as it engages, you will not comprehend anything that you hear from that point forward. If what was said is important, you will have to ask them to repeat it again. This will continue until you clearly experience and understand what is communicated.

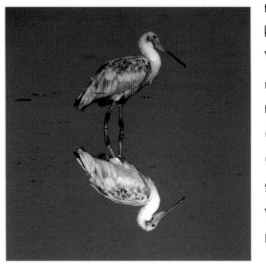

When consciousness is undisturbed in the present moment, it reflects things as they are—clearly. All meditation techniques, yoga or Qi-gong exercises are only trying to do one thing—go beyond the chatter or disturbance to the consciousness. Please be aware that yoga or Qi-gong exercises by themselves will not be effective if you don't know how to let them happen, because your expectations will disturb the process. I like to give an analogy of exercises as empty container (box) and consciousness (diamond) as the content. Without the diamond, the box is not worth much because it is only an empty box. When you are totally one with a movement, you will feel a million things as the consciousness (content) illuminates your body (the container). Yoga and Qi-gong exercises are the easiest way for you to experience this phenomenon.

In the last four chapters, we have identified several sources of disturbance:

1) Expectations and comparisons—the two main processes of the mind.

Managing Expectations and Comparisons

2) The lack of focus or the ADHD (attention deficit hyperactivity disorder) behavior due to the constant movement of the inner eye.

3) Too much talk and lack of listening.

You have also learned exercises to experience the state of silence and consciousness. All of these exercises combined together will systematically undo a lot of processes that you may have created in your brain. Your mind has become like an automatic machine; when you put in the ingredients (thoughts) it starts to process. The exercises in this book are designed to systematically disassemble the machine itself so that there are no automatic processes left. When all the gears are disassembled in your brain, if you get a thought, the machine does not exist, so no automaic process can happen.

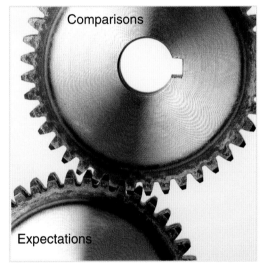

Comparisons

Expectations

It is all about efficiency. If you react to every thought or stimulus that comes to you, then where is the comprehension? However, if thoughts come into your consciousness and are carefully laid down in your being as components of a whole picture, you can be objective about your response. You will only say things when you have the whole picture or say things that you know because you have the facts. This will make your life very easy.

In continuing to understand the thoughts that we get, it will be good to understand why we have different durations for our thoughts. Not only will it enhance our understanding of them, but it will also show how to deal with them when they come into our consciousness. We will be able to organize our memory structures so that things don't pile up (information overload) until we are dealing with ten different thoughts at the same time with an inefficient allocation of energy.

Type A & Type B Thoughts

Two types of thoughts happen to everyone. I classify them as "Type A" thoughts and "Type B" thoughts.

Type A thoughts are everyday practical thoughts based on desire. They are caused by the energy moving in a million different directions because of our accumulated conditionings (past unconscious experiences). Type A thoughts don't occupy the consciousness for long periods of time, and they don't use much energy. An example of a Type A thought is opening your refrigerator and finding that there is no milk. A thought occurs that there is no milk and the next time you go to the store, you need to get some. Not having milk is a Type A thought.

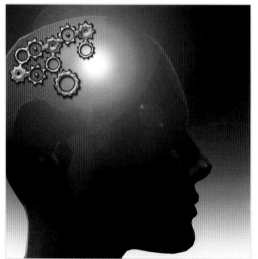

Another might be: "The kids need supplies for a school project." You make a list and buy them. Like Post-It notes, you use Type A thoughts to remember things, and discard them when done. Type A thoughts don't engage, possess or involve your consciousness.

However, some thoughts engage, possess and involve you for long periods of time. I call them Type B thoughts. When you have a Type B thought, you cannot feel anything else because it takes over. You do not have any comprehension about what you have eaten, what you are wearing or what you are doing. If you read something, you don't remember what you read. In the shower, you might not even remember if you used shampoo. In other words, you are not present, but are definitely engaged in some inner struggle. Your ego or psychological conditioning causes Type B thoughts and creates "virtual reality."

A Type B thought can be illustrated by imagining a situation: You and your boss are not getting along well, and one day things take a turn for the worse. Given the atmosphere in your company, you come to the conclusion that there is a good chance that you might get fired. Once this thought occurs to you, it divides your consciousness into two parts: seed thought and ancillary thoughts.

The "seed thought" is that you are going to get fired. All the "ancillary thoughts" are why you should not be fired. A whole list of your past achievements, why your boss is not a reasonable person or why he/she is racist and sexist, will be disturbing your consciousness. Thoughts will come like, "What will I do if I lose my job?" Your survival and aspirations are at stake. You don't even know if you are going to get fired. It is a hunch. You have assumed, and now have taken ten steps to avoid it. You have created your own virtual reality. The anticipation of the problem causes more turmoil than the problem itself.

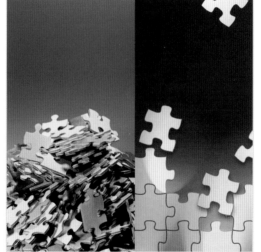
Information without consciousness is like a heap of puzzle pieces with no clear picture.

How do you know if you are having a Type B thought? If you are engaged for more than 30 seconds, you are having a Type B thought.

Impact on Our Consciousness

Say on a beautiful summer day you are walking barefoot in a park. While walking, you suddenly step on a thorn. Now you will have two types of walks: the one before (in balance) and one after the thorn (out of balance). Your immediate reaction would be to sit down and remove the thorn (the cause of pain). Once the thorn is removed, you find yourself once again in balance.

Now imagine a thought to be the thorn that enters your consciousness. As soon as it enters, it starts to disturb it. Instead of removing the thorn, you start to touch it, hoping to get a grip on it but you can't. It keeps going further and further into your consciousness, making things worse—creating a whole web of thoughts. Then, when it is too far gone, you give up on it and ask what you should be doing to live your life with the thorn still disturbing your consciousness.

What actually happens when you find yourself in the middle of a Type B thought or a stressful situation? Scientists and medical doctors have identified the following steps:

Step 1: Stress response originates in the brain: The hypothalamus, amygdala and pituitary glands go on alert as soon as they encounter a Type B thought. They release signaling hormones and generate nerve impulses that prepare the body to survive stress.

Step 2: The two opposites: A part of your mind keeps creating Type B ancillary thoughts that are perceived to be an immediate threat to your survival, while another part is fighting full-force to eliminate the threat. It is like pressing on the accelerator and the brake of a car at the same time—your car will overheat (inflammation) and blow the engine (heart attack).

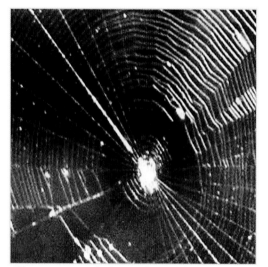

The center of the web is like a Type B seed thought.

Biologically speaking, your nerve cells release norepinephrine that tenses and constricts your muscles. This stiffness causes your breathing to become shallow, which means less oxygen intake. So your body intelligence kicks in, with your adrenal glands releasing epinephrine and cortisol so your heart and lungs work harder.

Step 3: The relentless damage: It is not outrageous to say that you may have an average of over 50 Type B-related thoughts on any given day. This could be one or two Type B seed thoughts and all the other attached, ancillary thoughts. Each time you get a Type B thought, your body has to go through the whole stress routine. Your body gets extremely stiff and strained and although it tries to loosen up from these extremes, a level of habitual muscle tension remains. This condition causes energy flow to break down, and leads to disease. We live and die prematurely in pain.

I know many people whose lives have come to a virtual standstill because they cannot get a break from their Type B thoughts; their conditioning keeps bringing the same unaware responses. This can lead to depression, anxiety, obsessive behavior, and other mental illnesses.

Relationship Between Type A and Type B Thoughts

Type A thoughts are caused by desire, and are energy-based. Type B thoughts are caused by fear and are the psychological interplay of fears and desires. Therefore, Type A thoughts are a superset that contains Type B thoughts. Desire is the source of all thoughts. Without desire, we cannot have fear.

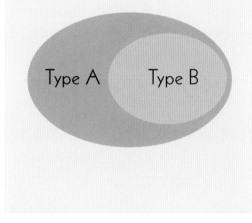

Techniques to go Beyond Type A and B Thoughts

Type A

Type A thoughts can be reduced and eliminated by doing the exercises shown in the first four chapters. When you have too many Type A thoughts, it is like a sand storm in your consciousness. Doing relaxed movements, taking a walk in the park, getting a massage or anything else that relaxes you will eliminate Type A thoughts.

Type B

Type B thoughts are based upon fear; they severely impact your consciousness, and need to be dealt with in a direct way. If you are a beginner who has not experienced silence or meditation, you might have a lot of Type B thoughts. Type B thoughts are the ones that engage your consciousness for long periods of time. The quickest, most effective and permanent solution to Type B thoughts is ACCEPTANCE.

Our response to a Type B thought is either fight or flight. If you think you have a large arsenal, then you will fight the Type B seed thought. Otherwise, you will try to run by suppressing your thoughts. In either case, you will lose. Neither fighting nor running is a good idea, because in both cases you are occupied with thoughts that drain your energy.

When you first discover that you are being engaged or possessed by a never-ending thought, remember, you are in a Type B situation. Rule of thumb: If a particular thought engages you for more than 30 seconds, it is a Type B thought. Given your past experience with Type Bs, you know very well where this is going to go—look for the seed thought.

In the example, the seed thought was that you would get fired. At this time, bring your total awareness to the seed thought and, unconditionally, without exception, accept it. Accept the thought that you are going to get fired. By your acceptance, you are not actually getting fired, but you are facing your fear of getting fired. The Type B seed thought is the thorn in your consciousness.

How to Identify a Type B Seed Thought

Look for two things: What are you fearing and what are you desiring? In the "getting fired" example, your fear is that you are going to get fired, and your desire is to not get fired. So your seed thought is the fear of getting fired. Accept your fears, no matter what they are, and you will be stress-free.

When you accept a Type B seed thought, these miracles will happen:

1) To accept a Type B seed thought, you naturally have to be aware of it. By becoming aware, the seed thought loses its steam, starts to die and ceases to control you.

2) With the seed thought gone, there will be no ancillary thoughts.

3) Each time that you get a Type B thought, you are unconsciously preparing for a war. Your body is always the scapegoat and must allocate a lot of energy to fight this war. With no war, only peace

exists and all the energy will be used by the body to rebuild.

4) If you apply this exercise of accepting the seed thought five to ten times in different Type B situations, you will have no recurrence of them. This is because you have eliminated the entire response process in your brain. If you do well with identifying and accepting the seed thought, then you are fully equipped to deal with any situation that comes your way. You know exactly what to do; after its 30 seconds of play are up— you are back to your silence again.

Things to Remember About Acceptance:

Acceptance of a Type B seed thought is the solution. In reality, the irony is that 99% of all Type B seed thoughts never come to fruition. In the "getting fired" example, it is only your hunch—it is possible that your boss may have had a bad day. You never evaluate the validity of a thought and yet you devote your entire energy to it without even questioning. You gamble with your energy all day long. Energy is the most rare and expensive thing that you have. To get a little bit of energy, imagine what you have to go through: have a job to earn money, buy and prepare food, eat and digest it, hopefully exercise, be stress-free and much more. For energy to happen in your body you have to have everything going right. However, you squander it without even thinking twice because you latch on to a Type B seed thought and it drains everything you have or will have. It is like some thief who has stolen your identity and is taking funds out of your credit card account.

It does not matter what kind of thought you may have: sexual, angry, jealous, perverted etc. You may say it is impossible to accept some of these thoughts because they go against who you think you are. Some of the thoughts can be very alarming and upsetting. Remember, they are your conditionings, which are things put into your consciousness without your being aware of it. With each layer of conditioning, your consciousness is further divided into pieces. Pretty soon there is no consciousness left. This is how we grow up—in darkness, without clarity, so we cannot see what lies ahead of us. Type B thoughts can happen at any time, without any notice; they catch you off-guard and then you go through the consequences. You might get a thought that you are running naked down Main Street in the middle of the afternoon, and the whole town is chasing after you. You might condemn yourself and contemplate getting help. However, if you understand that this is a Type B thought, you will avoid any unnecessary waste of energy. Type B thoughts are totally virtual.

So no matter what the Type B seed thought, your response should always be to become alert and totally accept it.

How Thoughts are Stored and Processed

Physiologically, we store all our information in different parts of the body through our nerves. Ayurveda (an ancient Indian science of living: see Chapter 9) says that thoughts or information are stored in a viscous liquid called tarpaka kapha. In

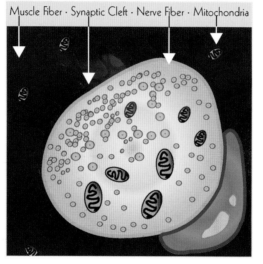

Muscle Fiber · Synaptic Cleft · Nerve Fiber · Mitochondria

between each nerve ending and muscle fiber, there is a space called the synaptic cleft or neuromuscular joint. Synaptic clefts are filled with tarpaka kapha making your whole body a storage house of information. If you lose your consciousness while information is being stored, it will remain in an unprocessed crystallized form—incomplete. This process is like a computer that loses all unsaved work if the power goes off abruptly. When you're under stress you may feel a burning sensation in your diaphragm or stomach because the tarpaka kapha (information) has not been fully processed.

How does the consciousness (power) failure happen in the body?

When the thought that you are going to get fired enters your consciousness, it gets written into a crystallized form because it needs to be consciously evaluated and resolved. However, instead of evaluating the validity of the thought, you act upon it as if it is true. Once you act upon an unevaluated seed thought, you lose contact with it and it will remain unresolved, creating chatter. Chatter is similar to pain; they both give information to us. Chatter gives information about the wounds in your consciousness, and pain gives information about the wounds in your body.

What happens when your consciousness is disturbed?
It is similar to losing electricity while toasting a piece of bread— it will be half done. You will have to repeat the toasting process for the required period of time. When you get interrupted by a thought, your consciousness focuses on dealing with it. If you are reading, then comprehension will stop because there is no consciousness flowing to reading, just like the toasting process stops without electricity. Without electricity, your bread is left cold and without your consciousness, your experience is left cold

and unclear. If you start and stop a toaster 20 times in five minutes your bread will never get toasted. If you get interrupted 20 times in a span of five minutes, you will have little or no comprehension.

The irony is that instead of bringing uninterrupted electricity to the toaster, you blame the toaster and say it is broken. In the same way, instead of bringing consciousness into your body, you find faults with the body. This solution will not work. The obesity problem in America and other developed nations is because of denial of the body and fixation on an ideal image. In finding faults with the body, you will miss your life. Will anything else matter if we miss our lives? Do we have an infinite number of days to live in this body?

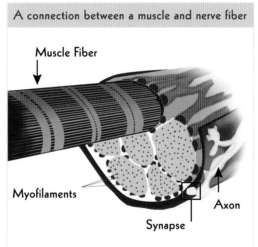

A connection between a muscle and nerve fiber

Muscle Fiber

Myofilaments

Synapse

Axon

Can chatter be helpful?
Your chatter keeps moving in circles around a particular seed thought that you have not resolved,

just like pain moves around a particular wound in your body. When we have chatter from many different seed thoughts and we don't know what to do, we try to drown them with drugs, food, or shopping to name a few ways. We start to live with chatter, like it is something normal, because everybody has it. Learning to listen as explained in the previous chapter is the only thing that is going to help. Thinking of it negatively and trying to shut it out will not be a permanent solution.

Is there a solution?
Bring your consciousness (awareness) to this crystallized part (Type B seed thought) and it will start to melt and diffuse. When you bring an awareness and

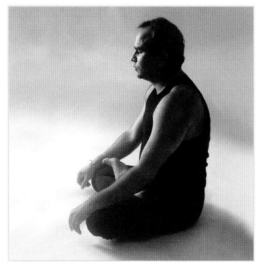

understanding to the seed thought, you will transcend it and heal. Lack of consciousness not only creates chatter but also causes imbalances (pain) in the body.

An Everyday Technique to Transcend Type B:
This technique can be done in the following simple steps:

1) Sit with your whole body still and your head straight for about 10 to 15 minutes.

2) Start to listen to any sound that might be present in your environment. While listening to sounds you may have thoughts that come into your consciousness. Listen to them with alertness.

3) If you have a particular thought that is presenting itself over and over again, then you probably have a Type B situation. Listen to that thought and find out what it is trying to say. In your awareness determine what is the fear and desire behind the thought.

4) Once the fear is identified as your seed thought, all you have to do is internally acknowledge it and accept it without any condition.

5) You will find that after you have totally accepted the thought in this way, it will never come back and bother you again.

What if this happens when you are at work? This technique can be done during the day when you may be at work, home or on the street. If you have a thought that is running over and over again in your head just stop whatever you are doing, close your eyes and look into the fear behind the thoughts. Once you have identified the fear and accepted it, it will be gone.

If you are new to the practice you may get involved with your thoughts easily. That is normal and OK. Practicing this technique for 15 days to a month diligently will show you its power in removing Type B thoughts. To become aware of the Type B seed thought is 90% of the success and the rest will happen when you unconditionally accept it.

The diagram given on page 89 can be used to identify the fears and desires behind a seed thought. This will make you more thorough in documenting the type of thoughts that you are experiencing. In the star, which represents the seed thought, write down a seed thought that you have identified. In the arrows pointing left, write down all the fears that you have experienced with the seed thought, and then do the same with the desires. The diagram is a tool to make your process of elimination efficient. Make copies of this diagram and use them. You may want to keep a binder of all the Type B thoughts that you may have had. This will help you see patterns in your fears and desires.

Why this Strategy Works?

The effectiveness of this technique lies in the fact that you have classified the thoughts into two categories: Type A and Type B based on the time they occupy your consciousness. When you do encounter a particular thought in your consciousness you know exactly what to do. You have a very clear decision-making tool; once you have identified the thought your solution is very clear. When you don't have a clear decision making tool you may end up giving more time to a Type A thought and no time to a Type B thought. This is not an efficient way to handle chatter.

When in the Real World...

You will have many more Type A thoughts than Type B thoughts. Even though Type A thoughts give practical information, they can disturb your consciousness when too many come in at the same time, especially when you need to focus. Type B thoughts will occupy your entire consciousness, period. Your daily practice from Chapter 3 is excellent for both Type A and Type B thoughts—understand and use the oil lamp example in whatever you do. It is the best medicine for reducing overall chatter from your consciousness. However, if you are dealing with a particular Type B issue, you can try these two steps to deal with them:

a) Look for your expectations and comparisons first, and deal with them directly as discussed in Chapter 1.

b) If the thoughts keep persisting in your head then look for your fears and desires associated with your seed thought. Accept the seed thought and be free from it.

If you have too many Type B thoughts at the present time, you may have to do this exercise a few times as well, but it will be worth it.

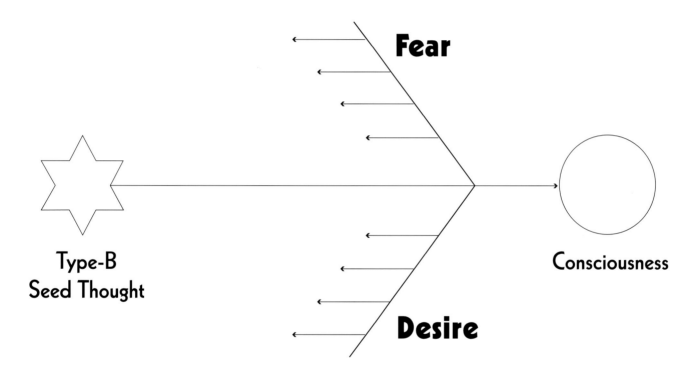

Fear

Type-B
Seed Thought

Desire

Consciousness

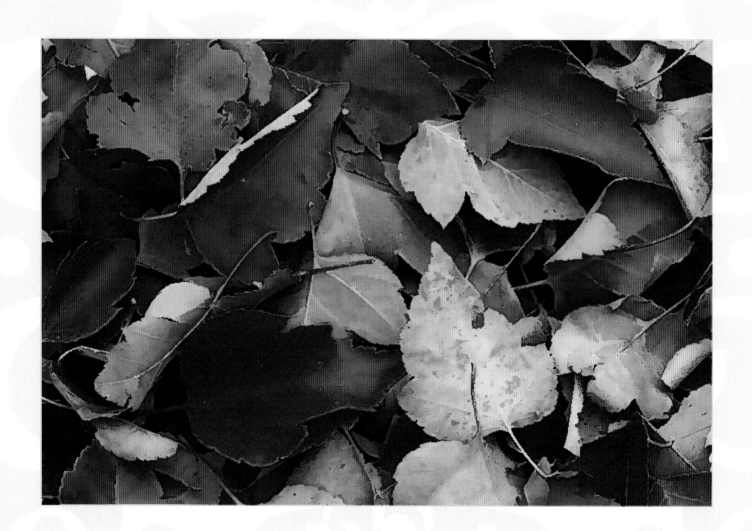

SPLENDOR of ended day, floating and filling me!
        Hour prophetic—hour resuming the past!
Inflating my throat—you, divine average!
        You, Earth and Life, till the last ray gleams, I sing.

Open mouth of my Soul, uttering gladness,
        Eyes of my Soul, seeing perfection,
Natural life of me, faithfully praising things;
        Corroborating forever the triumph of things.

Illustrious every one!
        Illustrious what we name space—sphere of unnumber'd spirits;
Illustrious the mystery of motion, in all beings, even the tiniest insect;
        Illustrious the attribute of speech—the senses-the body;
Illustrious the passing light! Illustrious the pale reflection on the new moon in the western sky!
        Illustrious whatever I see, or hear, or touch, to the last.

Walt Whitman Song at Sunset (Leaves of Grass)

Anything that you do, you can break down into three components. For example, say you have to get an injection at the doctor's office. The doctor prepares and gives you the injection in your right arm. The three components will be: The right arm, the needle (injection), and all the sensations (burning, pain, and discomfort) that happen from the prick. Another example would be eating an apple. The components would be: the apple, the chewing process or the body, and all the sensations (taste, temperature, texture) that you feel while eating the apple. Another simple example would be while you are walking. The three components would be: the road or the path where you are walking, your body or the walking itself, and finally all the sensations and experiences that happen to you while walking. Take a moment and break down reading this book into three components.

If only the three components existed, everything would be wonderful. However, very rarely in our lives are the three things in their purest form. There is always the influence of a fourth component—the disturbance. The fourth component consists of expectations, comparisons, analyses, manipulations, fears, desires, virtual reality, Type B and Type A thoughts. Let us revisit the examples above and see how the fourth component influences each of them. Even before the doctor gives you the injection, you may have thoughts in your head such as: "Oh, this is going to hurt badly," "I don't think I can watch this happen," or "Why am I doing this? Maybe I should run away." The entire process of the injection is not experienced, but lost in the mental chatter.

If you are not chewing the apple properly, or reading a book or talking with someone at the same time, you will find that you are not experiencing the apple. We have reduced eating into a mechanical phenomenon or a necessary evil. This type of eating habit deprives us of most the sensations and experiences of taste, so we find ourselves eating more, which leads to food addictions. Not chewing the apple properly leads to improper digestion and throws our body into a state of imbalance. The chatter or the fourth component deprives us of the experience.

Managing Expectations and Comparisons

While walking, if you are filled with expectations of reaching your destination within a certain time, you will probably not enjoy the walk very much. Your whole body will be tense, taking all the joy and fun out of your walk. The disturbance keeps you from experiencing the walk; you won't notice how you place your left foot or right foot, if you are stronger on the left side versus right side, does your breathing pattern change according to the walk? If you keep walking unconsciously for a long time, it can be a source of disease to your body.

A Simple Stretch

Let us use a simple stretch and break it down into three

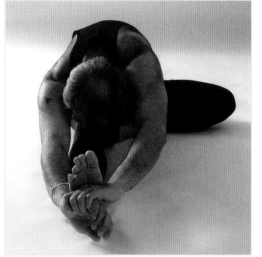

components: the body, movement of the left foot next to the right thigh and your head coming to your knees, and all the sensations and adjustments that your body makes to fulfill this stretch. Once again, while doing this stretch, if you have expectations on the outcome of this stretch, you will stiffen yourself and defeat the purpose of stretching.

If, by some miracle, the entire disturbance were removed, what would happen? You will be totally relaxed, and gently your head will come forward to the right knee and you will have a feeling that you could stay there forever. In addition, you will be able to see every little adjustment that your body makes. The information from every part of your body will be revealed in your consciousness such as: pain or discomfort in the hamstrings, calves, lower back, shoulder, or your breathing pattern. It is not possible to list all of the adjustments that your body is going to make or you will experience. Once the experience of pain or discomfort becomes clear in your consciousness, it will get processed and move or adjust your body ever so slightly, making all the difference in the world. It is like when all the pieces to a puzzle are put together and you see the final picture.

One thing you will also notice is that all of this can happen because you have no disturbance. With disturbance, none of this would be possible. In other words you will find out for the first time that things are perfect as they are and there is a lot to be learned from every simple thing in life. When we bring the fourth component or disturbance to it, we only make it worse. By clearly witnessing this phenomenon in your body, you will give birth to spirituality in your life. You will recognize that in everything you do, there is a divine conversation happening between the three components—this is the holy trinity. The holy trinity happens when the conversation between the body movement, the pain or discomfort from the movement and the consciousness is undisturbed.

Our problem is that we don't know that this divine conversation is happening within our body and around us all the time. We feel like we have to do a lot in order to connect with the universal consciousness. In our effort, we disturb it.

Reducing the Fourth Component

Remember that the fourth component is your ego. It is made up of all your conditionings: expectations, comparisons, fear, desire, analysis, Type A, and Type B thoughts. While doing anything, be mindful of the three components. As soon as you find that you are having chatter or making expectations, just realize it and you will find that it will lose its grip on you. The best way for the three components to come into sync is while you are doing your stretching practice as suggested in this book or DVD.

A Simple De-Cluttering Technique

Our brain has an interesting way of processing information; it cuts out all the empty space between objects that we see. For example, look around your living room you will find that you will see all the furniture and objects in the room, but you will never see the space within the room. The space within the room is completely cut out like it is not even there. The space in between the objects is the key because the space will always be there as objects come and go.

The Technique

Sit down on the floor or a chair, bring your palms together as shown in the picture. With your eyes open bring all your awareness to the space in between the palms. Once you become aware slowly move your palms about a foot and a half apart (as shown in the picture). Once again focus or remain aware of the space in between the palms. You will feel as though the space is expanding or

contracting. You will start to feel a certain sense of calmness descending upon you. As you remain with the space in between, you will be able to remain chatter-free.

After you have moved your palms side to side for at least three to four minutes move your palms in a different direction back and forth as shown in the picture. Once again the focus is on the space and not the objects in the space. With your palms moving back and forth you will find that the space is constantly moving and changing.

Why Is This Technique Important?

The key to this technique is that it takes all the brain focus/energy away from your thoughts and reroutes it to the space in between the thoughts. Once the

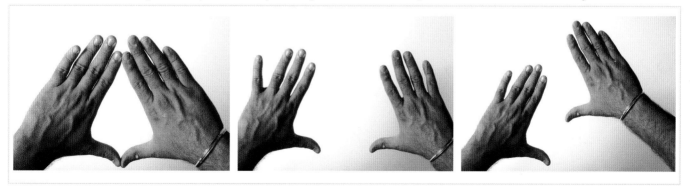

focus goes into the space in between the thoughts, your thoughts and chatter lose their steam and you get a break from them. In addition your virtual reality with the thoughts is broken or you are awakened from your fixation with thoughts. This technique, when done prior to the yoga/Qi-gong exercises, will help start the consciousness flow process through your body.

The flow process will feel something like this:
When you do the Qi-gong movement there will be times when you will find that you cannot consciously tell whether you are outside the body or inside the body. You will lose all identity to your ego that defines itself with the body. When you are in that state, you are in a state of oneness. This is your center. When this process happens, another process starts to happen: your body starts to get energized and you will feel a tingling sensation in between your fingers, your lower lip, arms, legs etc. This is your body's bio-electricity. In this state, the ultimate form of healing happens in your body. You will find that your entire skeleton is buzzing with energy and every pore of

your being is buzzing with energy. There are no words for this state; you will also notice that there are no thoughts that can pass through you. This is very significant because the consciousness that passes through you has discovered that you are not just your thoughts.

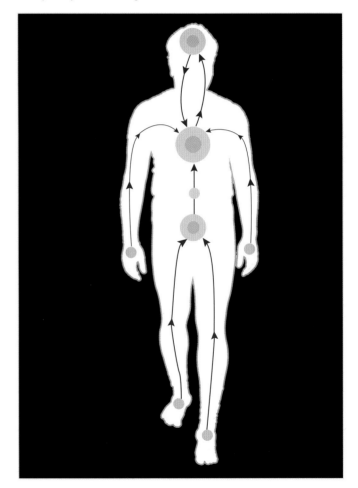

Managing

Expectations and Comparisons

In the Real World

These simple exercises are extremely powerful because they let you focus on the space and not on objects. When you do these simple hand movement techniques, you will find that you instantaneously relax and enter into a deep state of silence. I would recommend doing these exercises for five to ten minutes every day before your yoga/Qi-gong practice. Also, anytime you feel overwhelmed or stressed, these simple hand movements will bring you back to the center/consciousness. If you do these movements before you go to sleep, the quality of your sleep will improve as well.

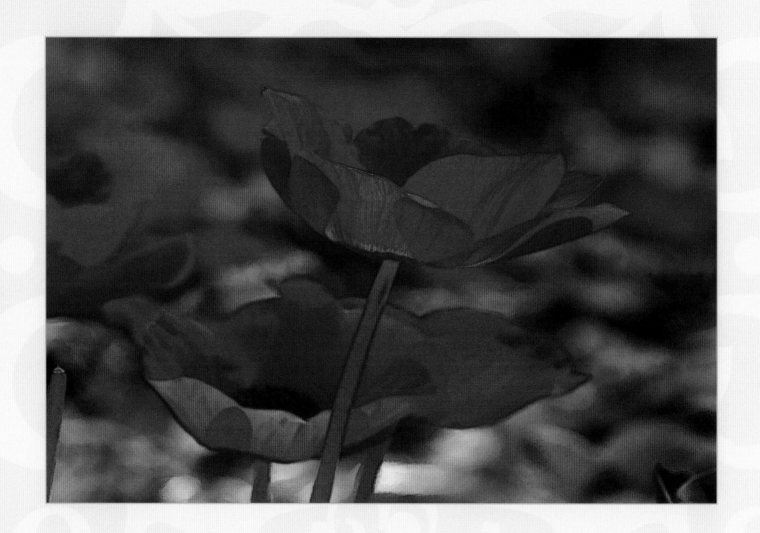

Children are living beings -
    more living than grown-up people
        who have built shells of habit around themselves.

Therefore it is absolutely necessary for their mental health
    and development that they should not
        have mere schools for their lessons, but a world
            whose guiding spirit is personal love.

Gurudev Rabindranath Tagore (mystical poet, Bengal, India)

One of the major problems that we face in today's world is the education of our children. Theoretically, we want to do the best for them to the best of our abilities. However, what happens due to our actions is often different from what we say we want. There are two reasons:

a) We have not defined clearly what it means to be educated. Do letters next to your name mean that you are educated?

b) Do we have adequate resources and training to help our child achieve his or her needs and aspirations?"

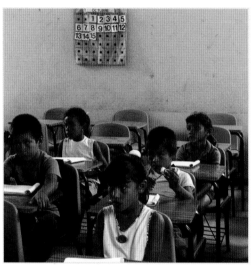

What Does it Mean to be Educated?

The main question to be asked here is, "What am I going to do with my education?" The usual answer is to get a job, make a living, have a career, and contribute to society. What about stress? Do we say that I want to educate my child so that he or she will be able to cope with stress better? In reality, our educational system has become a stress to our children. We set up expectations and goals for our children and then push them by comparisons to achieve. The downfall of having unrealistic expectations is discussed in Chapter 2. In many cases, parents project their own unfulfilled expectations onto their children, who naturally resent this. Their resentment then plays out like a movie for rest of their lives. Much love is lost and quality time wasted in this process.

Our entire life, and the society we live in, is based on consciousness. We differentiate between a dead person and a living person based on consciousness. We penalize people who act unconsciously in public (drinking and driving). We spend billions of dollars on the prevention of drug abuse in our society. Why are we spending so much money on prevention of drug abuse? Because drugs make you unconscious. When a loved one dies, we cry and mourn because they have become totally unconscious and have become incapable of consciousness again.

As a society, we are convinced that democracy is the best system in the world. This is because we believe that if all of the power goes in the hands of one person, and they lose their consciousness, then what will happen? Power and accountability is divided among several people on the premise that not everybody can become unconscious at the same time. Remember that unconsciousness can happen at any moment like in the example of when you are reading a book and suddenly a thought comes into your head. What is your ratio between being consciousness and unconscious? Can you read a book or do anything else without difficulty? Does your consciousness feel the silence when you are not doing anything, or is the radio perpetually turned on in your head?

There is not one place where we have connected education with becoming conscious, aware and alert. We have assumed that teaching math, science and English to our children in our schools will somehow translate into their becoming totally conscious, which is putting the cart before the horse. In fact, to be creative in math, science or English, one needs to be conscious and focused. It would be hard to imagine a rigorous mathematical proof or a beautiful poem that did not come from the depths of someone's consciousness. You will need focus and consciousness to get good at what is presented to you and not the other way around. Mathematics and science will not help take the chatter away from someone's life, it will only add to it.

We are confusing being informed with being conscious. We put labels on our cigarettes and show anti-drug advertisements hoping that by giving information, the people who read them will become conscious. This can also be seen in our religious practices that are based upon imparting information, whatever it might be. We believe that the stories and teachings that we share in our temples, churches, mosques and synagogues will translate into consciousness. This confusion between information and consciousness is the center of our education problem.

What Can Be Done?

We need to spend more time on consciousness in our schools and bring about a balance between information and consciousness. Think of consciousness as the foundation on which you are going to build a house of information. Without a foundation, the information that we give to our children goes into a pile and it is very hard to decipher the overall picture from it. Consciousness is like a light that helps you evaluate what comes into your being, where it needs to go and how it needs to be stored, so that when you need the information it is easily accessible. This process is efficient because you will avoid committing the same mistakes over and over again.

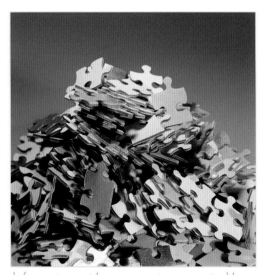

Information without consciousness is like a heap of puzzle with no clear picture.

If you are a schoolteacher or a student, try the following:

Alertness Routine:

1) Spend about 40 minutes each day (the equivalent of one class period) before the start of your school day to calibrate or tune into your consciousness. It is like gardening; before you are ready to sow anything in your garden, the ground needs to be prepared to receive what you intend to plant. Nothing will grow if your land is not prepared.

2) The first ten minutes just sit down, close your eyes and become alert to where the chatter is coming from. Is it more in your head, or coming from your jaw?

a) If it is coming from your head then let your whole body relax and take five deep breaths. For more information, review Chapter 3.

b) If it is coming from your jaw then just listen to what is being said. Like anything else, this might seem difficult at first, but after four to five days of practice you will get very good at it. If you still have a hard time, then close your eyes and listen to anything—it does not matter what you listen to as long as you listen. Once you become a listener, it will be impossible for you to have chatter coming from your jaw. To refresh your memory review chapter 4.

3) After the first ten minutes of practice, do all the preparation exercises given at the end of this chapter. Remember to relax while doing the exercises and let the energy move into the center of your brain as explained in Chapter 3. The oil lamp example is an excellent visual to remember while doing the exercises. Do the exercises for two to five minutes each.

4) In the last five to ten minutes just sit in silence. In less than a month, there will be very little chatter left in your consciousness. Also, you will be able to relax and enter your undisturbed conscious state quicker as you practice these exercises on a daily basis.

All the exercises and techniques are available on a DVD "Introduction to Consciousness." For quality, consistency and effectiveness, you can let the students view the entire DVD a few times to get acquainted with the forms and pace of the exercises. The idea is to be able to do the exercises with your eyes closed—it makes them much more effective.

What I am suggesting is not just theoretical; I have tried this practice in some of the most challenging schools in inner-city Cleveland. They are very effective if done consistently, in the right environment, where the teacher and the whole school have embraced the importance of remaining totally conscious.

Teachers are well aware of group dynamics in a class where they are exposed to a wide spectrum of students' abilities and challenges in a given day. Students' interests and their levels of consciousness range from excellent to poor. These techniques can only help because they will bring about a silence and focus that, generally, the students lack. Right away, the exercises will help the students that are already doing well. These students can then become good role models. The difference between a student in a good neighborhood school versus the one in the more challenged school is that of disturbance. In a more challenged school, the level of disturbance, both internal and external, is higher. Doing these techniques and exercises as a part of a daily curriculum will absolutely reduce their level of internal disturbance.

The Family Connection

The best gift that a parent can give to their child is for them to become fully conscious. In fact, that is what most conscientious parents do when they expose their child to different cultures, foods, and music. They want to make their children conscious of all that exists in the world.

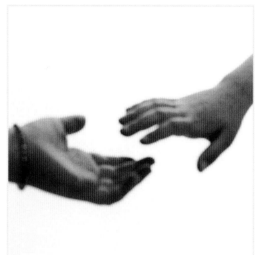

When there is little or no consciousness on the part of the child, the parent or both, things just don't work out right. The program outlined for schools can also be done at home. In addition, there are other exercises from chapter 9 that can be incorporated into your day-to-day practice.

Once you practice these exercises together, you will find you are having a lot of similar experiences that you can share as a family. This will develop a strong bond between all the family members. The irony is that you don't have to take expensive vacations or spend a lot of money to connect with your kids. Silence is the best way to connect with them. Unfortunately, we don't know how to do this. When we go to a mountain or a river or the ocean, we don't talk with them like we talk with another human being, yet we are so taken aback by their beauty. It is because when we are close to a mountain, we are slowing down and are silent. This silent communion with the mountain is what rejuvenates us. Creating an atmosphere of silence and communion in the house will make your own home into a vacation resort that you will never want to leave.

In today's world, we have over-medicated ourselves for everything; our solution is a pill. Unfortunately, this view creates more problems than it solves. This is a direct result of the lack of connection between the consciousness and the body. A case in point is ADHD (Attention Deficit Hyperactivity Disorder), now classified as a disease. Almost all diseases (except genetic diseases) can be linked to a certain lifestyle. Your body gets jittery when you eat food items that are high in sugar and caffeine. It is like trying to drive a car that can only go 55 miles per hour at 75 miles per hour. The jittery ride is not going to be much fun and you will ruin the car in the process.

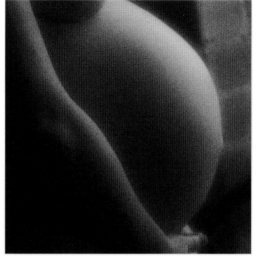

The outlined exercises and relaxation methodology will certainly calm the symptoms of this disorder and bring focus. In addition, all food items high in caffeine, sugar and carbohydrates should be avoided. A lot of blame can be put on the doctors, parents, drug companies and their lobbyists, and the government for all this, but it is you and your child who are paying the ultimate price.

It is in your best interest to do things that are natural for your child. Create an environment in your home or classroom where consciousness can happen and flow naturally.

Expectant Mothers

Doing the consciousness-enhancing exercises will have far-reaching implications. I had a wonderful opportunity to do Qi-gong and yoga exercises with two expectant mothers. One of them was my own sister. I am amazed at the similarity of their experiences:

a) Each baby was born healthy and without complications.

b) There were no problems with the deliveries.

c) Both babies cry very little and seldom fuss about anything except when hungry.

d) Each baby is silent and extremely alert.

All of these wonderful things are very significant, but my favorite one is "The baby is silent and extremely alert." When you bake a cake with all the required ingredients, the taste will be very good. However, if you forget or don't put the right ingredients into the mix, then the taste will not be the same. If you add silence and consciousness into your lifestyle while being pregnant it will impact your child as well.

What Exercises Can Be Done:
The following is a set of basic exercises that should be done everyday. There are over 11 Qi-gong exercises shown in the book, and you can do all of them. You may want to try and see which one takes you deeper into silence. If you have a lot of difficulty with chatter, then do the alertness routine.

Preparation Exercises
Stand upright, bare feet (if possible) with feet shoulder-width apart. Keep your body completely still and totally relaxed, and your eyes open in a soft gaze. Stand in this position for at least ten minutes. If you are silent, undisturbed, and relaxed, you will see your energy rising up to your head. It will make your whole body soft and supple.

Pay attention to the following:

- Practice your movements without any expectations or comparisons.

- In each stretch or movement, let the energy come into the center of your brain (see Chapter 3). It is the easiest way to come into your center and be chatter free.

- Let all of the movements and exercises be effortless like a bird flying and don't push or strain yourself. Move from one position to the next effortlessly.

- Stay in a particular position until you completely disappear in it.

At the end of each session, depending on how you feel, you can lie down.

Lotus Position (Padmasana)

Keep your eyes open and sit or stand. Looking straight ahead with soft eyes, be still. Stay in this position for at least ten minutes. Don't move or look for anything; simply sit or stand without any expectation. You are doing this for no particular reason-just doing it.

It is not absolutely necessary to sit in this position—being comfortable and relaxed is.

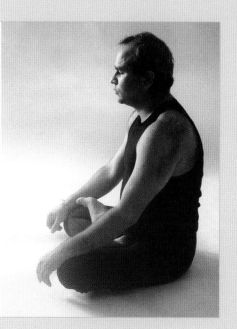

Qi-gong Rocker

Sit with your eyes closed (sit on a chair if you cannot sit on the floor). Place your palms next to your hips and bend your elbows. Slowly move your body back and forth from the lower spine. If you can imagine that you are doing this movement sitting in a swimming pool or ocean it will help.

Keep rocking your body back and forth gently without any expectations. You are not worried about the fact that you may be doing it wrong.

Keep moving for the next two to three minutes.

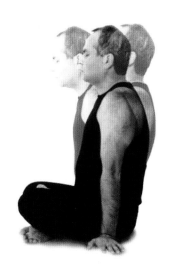

Qi-gong Head Movement

With your eyes closed and back straight, gently bring your head down until your chin touches the space between your collarbones. Then gently lift and move your head all the way back until it can go no further. Hold it there for few seconds and gently come down to the center. Then move your head all the way to the left and then to the right. Then bring your head to the center. Remember no expectations or comparisons about these movements.

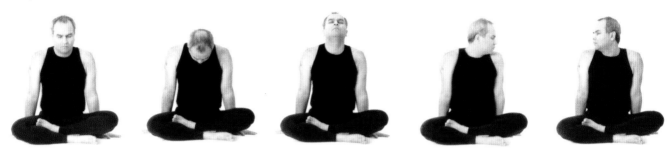

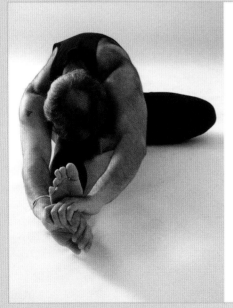

Janu Sirsasana (Head on Knees)

Without breaking the silence, bring your left foot out and your right foot next to your left thigh. Slowly start to move your chin towards your left knee while keeping your knee straight. Feel like you are pouring into this form. Stay in this position for at least two to three minutes. As always, with any stretch, you are ready to move to the next only when you have become relaxed in the form.

Change sides and bring your left foot next to your right thigh, keeping your right knee straight. Gently lower your chin towards your right knee. No expectations, and no comparisons to the other side. Feel the stretch coming from the lowest part of your spine. Stay in this form until you have become totally relaxed.

Managing Expectations and Comparisons

Sitting Lower Spine Twist

Softly and easily, place your left foot on top of your right thigh. Place your left arm behind your spine and place your right palm over your left knee. Feel the stretch in the back of your body and lower spine. Keep your eyes closed and stay in the stretch until totally relaxed.

No expectations or comparisons.

Change sides, repeat the exercise and stay in the form for three to four minutes. Once you are able to stretch fully, it will be very effective in letting the energy flow from the base of your spine to your head.

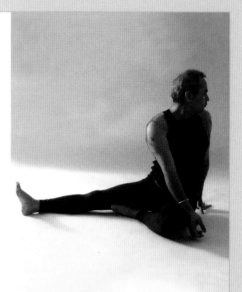

Seated Triangle (Upavistha Konasana)

Move your legs apart as far as they can go. While keeping your knees straight, move your chin towards your left knee and stay there as long as you can. Then gently move your head to the other side and bring your chin towards your right knee. Keep your knees straight and stay there as long as you can.

Then gently come out and bring your chin forward and go as far as you can without straining. Keep your eyes closed and body totally relaxed.

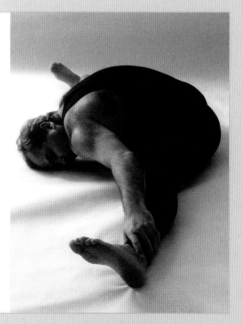

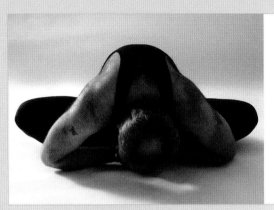

Baddha Konasana (Restraint Angle Stretch)

Bring both soles of your feet next to each other. If this feels too tight then bring your left foot over your right leg. Do the best you can, even if this feels tight as well. Bring your head forward, stretching from the lowest part of the spine. Stay in this form until you are totally relaxed.

This stretch may be hard to do if you are a beginner.

Body Energizing Qi-gong Movement

You can do this exercise either standing up or sitting down. Move your arms up and down gently (one at a time, as shown in the pictures) without any expectations or comparisons. Move them for at least three minutes.

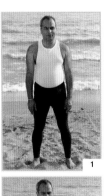
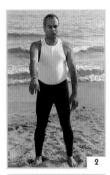
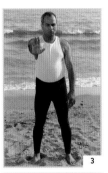
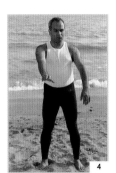
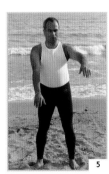
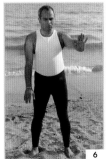
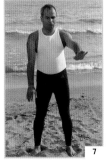
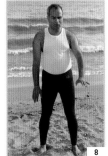
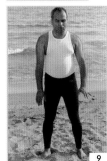
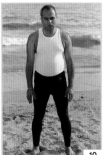

Managing Expectations and Comparisons

Becoming-One Qi-gong Movement

Let your arms rise up to the side without your doing. It should feel like someone is lifting them up for you. Keep moving your arms up and down (as shown in the pictures) for the next three to five minutes. Slowly and gently.

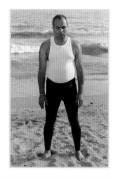 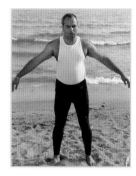 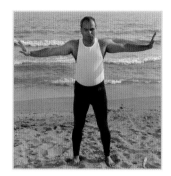 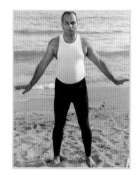 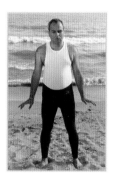

Body Balancing Qi-gong Movement

Bring both of your palms facing upwards below your navel. Gently let your palms rise up like someone is lifting them up for you. When your palms pass your heart center turn them around and let the palms start to flow downwards until it crosses over the navel. Repeat the movement for two to three minutes gently.

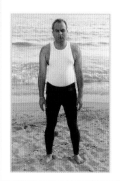 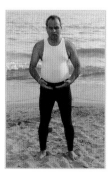 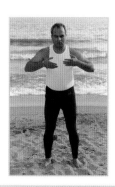 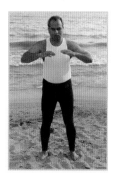 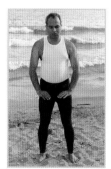 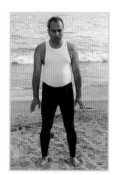

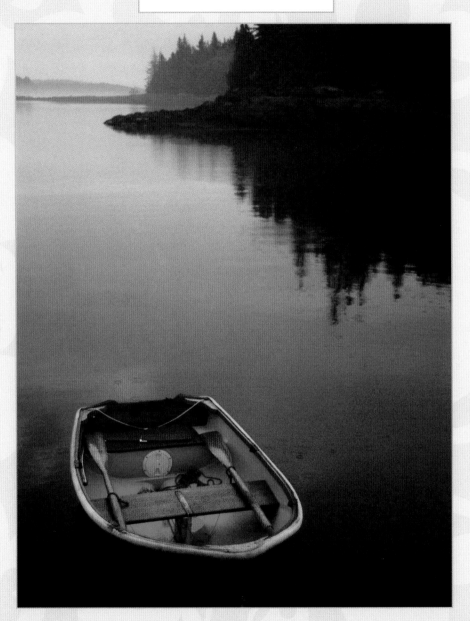

Perfect illustration of balance:

The still water represents the undisturbed
reflective state of consciousness.

The empty boat on the still pond signifies
the balance between the body and the consciousness.

The boat/body is empty of the disturbance
due to the mind and the two unused oars indicate

Lack of fear and desire.
No expectations and no comparison.

The power of expectation cannot be felt more clearly than in both amateur and professional sports. The underlying drives in any sport are expectations and comparisons. Look at professional baseball. We have statistics for each and every aspect of the game: how many home runs a player has hit, how many times a particular player has been struck out without scoring a run, and so on. There is no room for error. The checks and balances are in place on every minute-by-minute play and you are always under the microscope. The problem is that now, if you are a professional athlete, you have to fulfill not only your expectations but also those of the entire world. Sometimes, there is no room given to a faltering athlete to regain their focus and strength. A case in point is Tiger Woods, who has not been able to do as well in the early few months of 2004 as he has in the past. He clearly pointed out to a reporter that the media (world) does not let him forget anything and brings up the past, which seems to impact his game now.

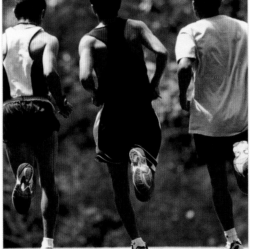

The entire field of sports is run on one thing: focus. This one thing will differentiate your performance from one event to the next. Focus is total conscious alertness. It is a state where there is no disturbance to your consciousness of any kind—no chatter. Focus not only impacts your score, but above all, it affects your whole life. You will be injured easily and have a hard time healing properly and quickly if you lack focus. When you are focused, your muscles, bones and all the cells of your body are relaxed. The energy intake and expenditure is at the optimum level. You are not wasting energy on things that take you away from what you are doing right now. In such a state, in whatever you are doing, you will feel a sense of fulfillment that is priceless; a "runner's high," which is a phenomenon that a few long-time runners have had the good fortune to experience. This phenomenon happens when you are running with total focus for 15 to 20 minutes—all of a sudden a burst of energy comes into you and you feel like you can go forever.

In stress, the flow of conscious energy through your body is disturbed, which means that the end point where you need the energy is not getting anything. Imagine a garden hose. If the entire 20-foot-long garden hose has a hole every two to three feet, and water is running through it, what do you think will happen towards the end where you need the water? You may not have enough for the type of work you want to do. Each hole in the garden hose will shoot out water in places where you don't need it and the water is wasted. This water hose is like the energy channel in your body. The holes in the energy channels can be translated into the chatter and stresses that drain your energy. The energy drains out of the channels and like a flash flood, overloads anything on its path—organs, bones, tissues, or muscles. This overload of energy in certain parts of the body is the cause of inflammation, which in turn, causes other diseases.

Paralysis by Analysis

Sound familiar? This expression can be applied to practically anything in life. Once you get into the maze of your mind, then there is no telling how long it is going to be before you come back to the present. This expression is very close to all golfers. Golf is an interesting game because it teaches you personal responsibility in a hurry. The ball does not move on its own, and how focused and connected you are to your body will determine how you are going to do on a course. No wonder a lot of business executives take up golf. At some level, it must be fulfilling their desire for focus.

Focus and analysis are opposites. In focus, there are observations and no analysis. Imagine that you walk into a dark room and you have no idea what is there. You touch something and start to create a mental picture of what you are touching. You are analyzing what you are touching because you cannot see. Now, if by a stroke of luck, you find the light switch and flip it on, all of a sudden you don't need to analyze anything. You don't look at a chair or a table or a lamp and analyze it; you know what it is and use it when required. When you are in darkness (due to chatter) you have to analyze; there is no other way for you to know. However, if there is light of undisturbed consciousness, no analysis is necessary—only observation. No analysis would imply no paralysis. This is true for any sports or any situation you might be in.

Focus in Team Sports

It is hard enough for one person to focus; imagine what happens when several players in a team play against another team. With focus, a natural rhythm starts to happen among all of the team members. It is like they start to speak some mysterious language and communicate in silence, synchronizing their actions. Each player knows where the other players are and they are well aware of their parts. This is awareness, which is a much deeper level of focus. The team members are able to see things in "real time" and adjust their game immediately, not the next day in their conference room. If the basis of a team is on focus it will naturally bring about a rhythm that will be hard to lose. This rhythm will not only bring the team members closer, but it will also lift the focus or joy of the people who are watching. If you watch a drunk person walk, you won't feel balanced; however, when you watch a circus acrobat, your own sense of balance is improved, no matter how short-term. All in all, there will be a consistency in the team's performance, which is essential for any group that wants to grow and make meaningful changes.

Creating an Environment and Not Expectation

An expectation is a goal that we create for ourselves and that drives us. Expectations will draw you back into the dark room where you will have to do analysis and pay the price by paralysis. This is a trap. You will pay the price, if you even go close to having expectations. There is no power in this world that can save you if your life is run by expectations. You cannot cheat either. It is like walking on a razor's edge. Learning to live without expectations may take a few days of practice, but the payoff is huge because if you can walk on the razor's edge, you can walk anywhere, anytime and any day.

Create an environment where focus can happen. Work on things that will bring about focus individually and see how they work for a team. Put all your eggs into the basket of creating the environment for excellence to happen. Like when you sow a seed, you are creating an environment, but you are not the creator of the plant or the tree. It is not in your hands. You cannot claim it. Just be happy that you had the great opportunity to sow a seed and watch the miracle of a tree or a plant growing.

What is the Solution?

To remove the processes within your body and mind that create chatter or disturbance. All the techniques discussed in the first five chapters help you become aware of these processes and give you ways to remove them. The expectations and comparisons that we unconsciously make over and over again will create more holes in your energy channel than anything else. Virtual reality will guarantee that these holes don't close easily.

Process and Instances

In the world of quick fixes, you are more geared towards instances and not to the process in the long run. This is very harmful, unfulfilling and expensive. To illustrate the difference between a process and an instance, imagine that you are sitting in a boat with a hole. Water gushes in and your boat is sinking. Since you are not sure exactly where the hole is, you are unable to plug it. Luckily, you have a small bucket that you use to dump out the water. This takes away the immediate threat of drowning, but the process of water leaking through the hole still continues. This is exactly how we handle stress and try to bring focus. We do it each bucket at a time because it makes immediate sense, but in the long run you miss important things in your life. All you know is how to dump the excess water out, and you know very well that you cannot stop. The water (stress) still keeps filling in the boat (body).

The only way you are going to be focused and stress-free is if you find the hole in the boat and plug it. This is what I call fixing the process. If you fix the process, you will be done with the stresses and problems originating from it for good and there will be no coming back. You will break the stress cycle:

1) The origin of chatter through a thought.
2) Short-term solutions to get beyond stressful thoughts.
3) The work of undoing the impact of stress on the body (short and long-term).

Focus, Flexibility, Endurance and Strength:

Focus

To bring about a clear focus, incorporate these three things in your life:

a) Go beyond the game of Expectations and Comparisons. They create more chatter and disturbance than anything else.

b) Do your everyday practice of deep stretching and energy movement exercises. These will ensure that the energy comes to its highest form without being blocked or dissipated in the middle. Remember the water hose example and the impact of leaks on its effectiveness.

c) Work on dissolving your virtual reality and you will naturally become focused. Find which fears and desires create virtual reality in you; this will ensure that your focus is not temporary but long term. Understanding virtual reality and its impact will help you cut away destructive and stressful thoughts easily.

Flexibility and Endurance

Yoga and Qi-gong exercises will not only build focus, they will also build your body by increasing flexibility and endurance. To understand how a higher level of flexibility and endurance can be attained, you have to understand what your body is made of. In this section, we will focus on what impact the exercises mentioned in this book have on your muscles. A human body has three types of muscles:

1) Skeletal (voluntary) muscles are attached to the skeleton and work when your brain gives a voluntary electrical signal to the muscle to contract. Your hamstrings, quadriceps and other such muscles fall into this category.

2) Smooth muscle is found in many systems including your digestive system, blood vessels, and bladder. Smooth muscles have an ability to stretch and maintain tension for long periods of time. They are also called involuntary muscles because you don't have to think about them; your nervous system controls them automatically. For example, when you eat food your stomach expands, and the muscles in your stomach automatically contract when the food is digested.

3) Cardiac muscle is found only in your heart, and its big features are endurance and consistency. It can stretch in a limited way, like smooth muscle, and contract with the force of a skeletal muscle.

How do they work?

Slow, deep stretches work on all three muscle types. As an illustration, let us use the "Intense Side Stretch"

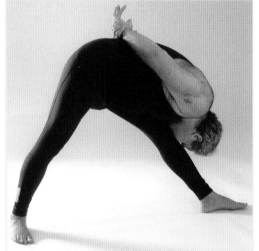

to see what actually happens while doing it. The picture illustrates the stretch.

With your legs between two and three feet apart, place your left foot facing forward, and your right foot at a 45 degree angle. Clasp your hands behind your back. Bring your face down to your left knee, close your eyes and relax. Stay there for two to three minutes and then switch sides. You will be able to feel the impact of this particular stretch even if you are not able to bring your face to your knee.

Did you notice?

When your legs extend apart and your face touches your left knee, you are putting a maximum amount of pressure on your left hamstrings and the muscles in your left leg. It will also stretch the outside muscles on your right legs such as the tensor fasciae latae, vastus lateralis, and the iliotibial tract. Your trunk comes close to your leg, putting intense pressure on the entire digestive system. Remember, all of this happens while your body is relaxed, so the muscles and other blood vessels are dilated (opened) for a full stretch. Your upper body faces downwards so that all of the blood flow goes to the head, heart and lungs, and is also exercised by the pressure against the leg. Your brain, pituitary, pineal, thyroid glands—and all the major glands of the body are getting the maximum amount of blood supply.

If you are aware and alert while doing the movements and the exercises as shown, you will be able to tell similar things about them. This awareness will develop an appreciation for your body, bring attunement and build tremendous flexibility.

Strength

As you use your muscles while exercising or going about your daily business, they get shortened and tight. Think of your muscles as big rubber bands that expand when needed and contract when their purpose or need is over. By constantly using the muscles in the body they naturally shorten and lose their elasticity. With the major muscles less able to move, all the pressure will be put on small delicate muscles in other parts of the body. For example, problems with the lower back are not just due to the weakening of the lower back muscles, but also from the tightening of the hamstrings and other leg muscles. When the hamstrings are tight and don't move, the pressure transfers to the lower back muscles which are not designed to withstand it, so they tear and unleash pain and suffering. Over time, the shortening of muscle fiber can cause ligament damage or joint hyper-mobility among other things. Deep stretching is the only antidote to the shortening of the muscles.

When a muscle group is put under force, the myofilaments (muscle fibers) shorten in response. When this force is removed, the muscles relax and come back to their original length. Energy is stored in your muscles during this sliding process, giving your muscles more power. Therefore, to increase strength and power, the muscle has to rest at its greatest length. All the exercises shown in the book encourage exactly that.

All of the information given here can be applied to any team, organization or company.

If you follow the directions on remaining focused and doing the exercises for two to three months, **you should see a tremendous positive shift in your life.** The suggestion can be done individually or as a team. In a team environment, there can be more support and sharing of experiences. **The good thing about working on your health is that the payback is immediate.**

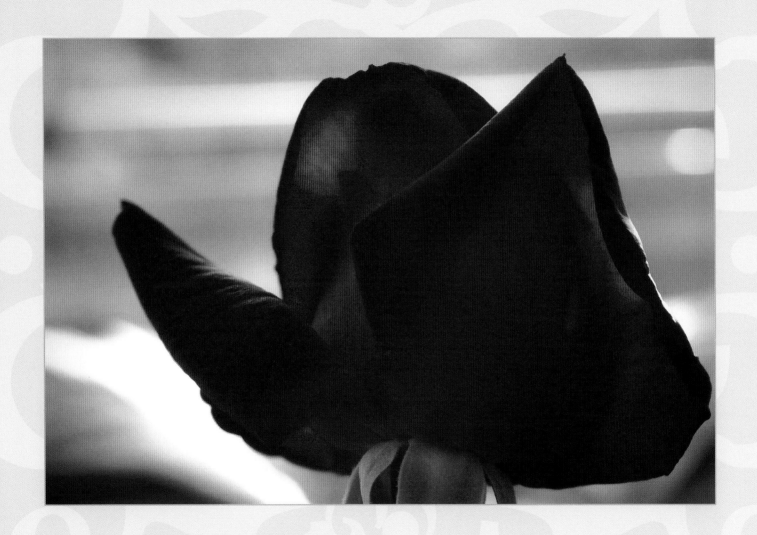

"This we know,

　　　the earth does not belong to man;
man belongs to the earth.

This we know.

　　　All things are connected like the blood
which unites one family.

Man does not weave the web of life—
　　　he is merely a strand in it.

Whatever he does to the web,
　　　he does to himself."

Chief Seattle, 1854

To understand the construction and functioning of a human body, it will be helpful to understand the construction and functioning of a house. A house has to be built based on climatic conditions. A modern house will have several distinct spaces such as a kitchen, living room, bedroom, dining room, bathroom, basement, and closets. It might also have heating and cooling, drainage, electrical and ventilation systems. Some parts to this house have to remain dry (living room, basement, kitchen), some need to have water (bathroom) and your kitchen has to have stove and heating appliances. Some parts of the house can remain cool (basement) while other parts need to be warm and comfortable (living room). In an ideal house, things function as they should.

To build a house, you need concrete, wood, insulation, electrical wires, systems for cooling or heating, and kitchen equipment. Similarly, your body is made up of plasma, blood, muscles, fat, bones, bone marrow, nerve tissues, connective tissues and sperm/ovaries. In both constructions, different spaces have different functions: Parts of

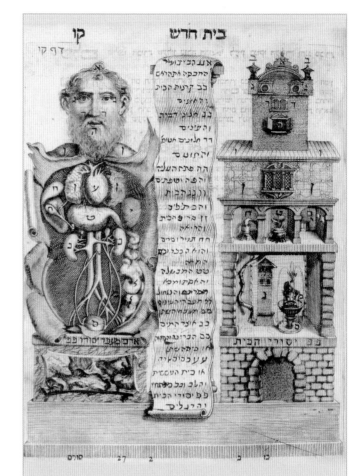

Toviyah Kats (ca. 1652-1729) This illustration from a Hebrew encyclopedia pairs the interior of a human interior with the interior of a house, a visual metaphor: the organs, like rooms in a house, have different functions. Kats, one of the first Jews to study medicine at a German university, completed his degree at Padua and served as court physician to the Ottoman Sultan. Source U.S. National Library of Medicine.

your lungs need to be dry, while your stomach can get hot, and your eyes and the cartilage in your knees need to be wet. Just as the living room is dry, parts of a kitchen can get hot and bathrooms are capable of getting wet.

As the owner/manager of the house, you have to keep up with its wear and tear. If you are aware and don't let things fall apart, you will enjoy the house comfortably. If water leaks in your kitchen, you tend to it before it reaches your living room or basement. Your house also has to be capable of sustaining stresses such as rain, heat, cold, earthquakes, tornadoes, mice, or bugs.

In the same way, your consciousness is the owner/manager of your body. If the owner is unconscious about what is happening, and there is a problem, nothing will be done. For example, when you overeat you find that it is very hard for you to move; you feel sleepy and have low energy. Somewhere within you, the manager was not conscious enough to say, "Let us stop now and not eat any further because the body does not have the ability to digest so much food." If you overeat repeatedly, you will gain weight and stress your whole body.

Often the consciousness or manager is unable to institute the changes to correct this imbalance. With no sign of management, everything starts to happen randomly or by accident. Then diseases can enter and make your body their permanent home because there is no relationship between your conscious-ness and your body. The goal of this chapter is to strengthen this relationship between your body and consciousness.

What does it mean to be healthy?

Foundation

To build any structure, you must have a firm, sturdy foundation. If it is faulty, sooner or later it will col-lapse. A human body is a structure that is constantly moving in many dynamic ways—you jump, walk, climb, crawl, lie down, get up, sit down, spin or twist. This makes it even more important to have a good founda-tion.

The way you stand on your feet is the foundation of your body. If you walk or stand putting too much pressure on the outsides of the soles, you will very likely have hernias and problems with your knees. If you put too much pressure on the insides of the soles you will have no arch, causing many types of abdominal problems and back pain. If you have a large stomach, you may be walking on your toes because your body is pulling you forward and if you have a weak back, shoulder or leg muscles, you will walk on your heels. Either way, you don't use your whole foot. Ninety-nine percent of all people don't use their entire foot to stand or walk—this includes well-trained yoga and Pilates practitioners. The main causes of these different types of imbalanced walks are psychological (stress), food habits and the type of training that we do with our bodies.

I have been to many races for charitable causes and am surprised to see that only five to ten percent of the runners do any type of stretching before they start. Imagine someone unknowingly putting a lot of pressure on the outside sole of his or her foot while running a distance of five to ten kilometers. They will make their body worse than ever before.

Four Types of Imbalanced Walks

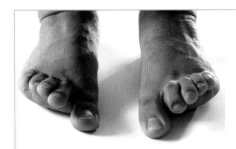

This picture shows too much emphasis put on the inside of the foot, essentially having no arch at all (flat feet), also known as pronation. This not only impacts the way you walk, but it can also be the origin of all types of back and abdominal problems. This problem happens when the muscles in the inside of your legs get weak.

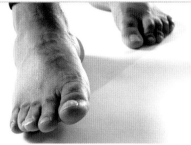

Most people have a type of walk where due to imbalance, only the heel and outside of the foot is used in walking or standing, also known as supination. This type of walk is the cause of most knee and hip-related problems. Each step you take with this type of alignment is essentially flexing your knees and hip bones on the outside causing the imbalance.

Osteoarthritis (arthritis of the knee) is due to this type of walk. Many other types of abdominal and back diseases can be traced back to this walk. This type of walk happens because the entire muscle structure on the sides of the body has become weak. Most people who have this type of walk will have a hard time doing side bends.

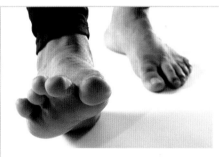

This type of walk implies using your heels to walk. Generally people who walk this way have a loud walk like they are thumping the floor. This walk is the main cause of all types of back problems. When you walk on your heel you are causing an imbalance between the upper and lower body. The point of stress is at your hips, especially your hip socket. When you hit your heel on the floor, your lower body is pushed backwards at the hip socket. Doing this automatically lunges your upper body forward. This then becomes so fragile that one day you try to lift something heavy and make the imbalance worse. That is, you pull the upper body forward from the lower half thereby displacing certain vertibrae in the spine—especially between L1 to L5. Once this happens, any type of back pain is possible.

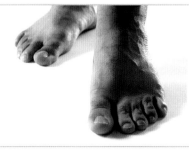

If you have a foot problem and no balance, you are probably walking on your toes. People who have weak muscles in the front of their body have this problem. If you are overweight or carry too much weight in the front of your body, you probably walk on your toes. This walking will cause many types of foot problems, not to mention strain on your back and knees.

How to bring your body into an alignment

Evaluate your stance and walk:

With bare feet, slowly walk 20 feet without stopping. While walking, pay attention to how you place the soles of your feet on the floor. Which part of the sole touches first and which is second? Next, see if you do the same thing with both feet. Make a clear note of what your right and left foot does. Then, stand straight with your eyes closed and watch how you stand. Do you put more pressure on the outside, inside, back or front of your feet?

Whichever side you put more emphasis on, know that side is weak and out of alignment. For example, if you put too much emphasis on the outside soles, the muscles on the outside of your legs and body are weak and need to be stretched and strengthened. If you are losing the arch of your foot by putting too much emphasis on the inside sole, the muscles on the inside of your leg are weak and need to be stretched and strengthened. The same goes for the front and the back.

Once again remember that whichever side you are putting more emphasis on while standing or walking, your body is weak on that side.

These six exercises will bring your body into total alignment. They have to be done in the given sequence. If you leave one of them out, your balance is going to be off. In many classes only standing or sitting exercises are taught, or only certain parts of the body are exercised on a given day—a sure way of throwing your body off-balance. These six exercises should be done every day in addition to any other exercises shown in the book. If you feel that you are weaker on one side, do an extra set to bring that part into balance. For example, if you are putting too much emphasis on the outsides of your feet, then do an extra set of side bends and side twists.

Managing Expectations and Comparisons

If you are planning to do these exercises on a daily basis, I recommend that you buy a new pair of flat shoes and discontinue using your old shoes. The soles of your shoes will be worn out in the imbalanced pattern of your walk. So when you start to correct the imbalance by doing the exercises and yet still wear your old shoes, you are going to feel discomfort.

1) Standing forward bend

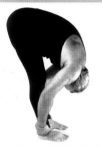

Keeping your jaws totally relaxed and your knees straight, bring your head down to your knees. Your focus should be on relaxing your jaws and your body. Stay there for at least three to five minutes and let your thoughts merge into silence. You will see that whenever your jaws are relaxed you have no thoughts. Seeing this connection is key for your mind to change and not be a source of disturbance.

2) Back bend

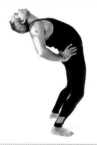

With your mouth slightly open, jaws relaxed and your palms behind your lower back let your head and upper body come as far back as possible. Don't overstretch yourself and stop wherever your consciousness finds a limit to your stretch—no expectations and no comparisons. Stay in this pose for at least three to five minutes.

3) Side bend

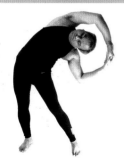

With your jaws relaxed, bring both of your palms together above your head and face upwards. Gently move your body to the left going as far as you can. Your entire focus should be on your jaws and relaxing them. You will find the more your jaws are relaxed the deeper your stretch is. Stay in this posture for two to three minutes and gently let your body move to the other side. Once again, stay in this posture for two to three minutes—coming out only when your consciousness is ready. Enjoy the silence.

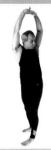

With your mouth slightly open and jaws totally relaxed, bring your palms together over your head facing upwards. Gently move your whole body from the lower spine to the left. Stop, wait and relax when you cannot go any further. Stay in this relaxed position for at least two to three minutes. Move to the other side only when you body gets the directions from the silent consciousness. Feel your body come alive.

5) Side split

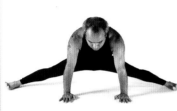

With your jaws relaxed and feet apart, bring your palms to the floor. Gently let your feet slide to the sides as far as your body can handle. This is the best exercise to see the relationship between relaxed jaws and relaxed body. You will be able to stretch deeply if you keep your jaws relaxed. In fact, anytime you feel discomfort you will find that your jaws are stiff and you probably are engaged in some internal chatter. When this chatter dissolves and all the energy flows into the body, the stretch becomes a door to experience blissful state of consciousness.

6) Strength and balance

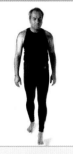

This stretch is a form of meditation technique. Standing upright with your jaws slightly open and totally relaxed, bring your left foot forward and place your left toes in front of your body. The entire weight of your body is placed on your right foot while your left toes give it balance. Stay in this posture for at least two to three minutes and then gently let your body change sides by bringing left foot back and right foot forward.

All the exercises should be done with your eyes closed once you become familiar with them. In the last stretch you may want your back away from a wall about two inches. The wall can give you necessary support when needed. As your body starts to balance, strengthen and become conscious, you will be able to stay in this posture for hours without moving. This will happen

After about a week of doing the exercises, you will find that you are walking more centered and standing upright. You are placing your foot flat on the floor each time you walk like any animal that places its paws very deliberately. Over a period of time, as your body gets into a further alignment, you will find that you feel a sense of warmth under your feet when you walk, like someone has lit them on fire. You will also find that your walk is simple as though you're gliding and there is absolutely no pressure on your knees. If you have calluses or other deformities on the soles of your feet, they will start to heal and wither away.

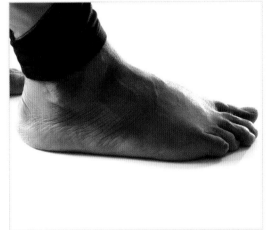

A sense of grounding and balance happens when the entire foot is placed on the ground.

Construction

Consciousness: the first step

A human being has three components: body, mind and consciousness. To understand the relationship between the body/mind/consciousness it will be helpful to use the example of turning on a light bulb in your house. You have four basic things: the bulb, wire, switch and electricity. The bulb and the wire are the body, the switch is the mind, and the electricity is the consciousness. The key is the switch (mind). If the switch is malfunctioning or disconnected, it will make it impossible for the electricity to flow to the light bulb. The same is the case with the mind; if it disturbs the flow of consciousness into the body, the body will have no energy. The sole problem is the switch because if you are alive, you have both body and consciousness. It is the faulty mechanism of the mind/switch that is causing the imbalances.

In Western medicine, only in the last few decades has the body/mind relationship gotten some attention. However, there is no understanding, formal training or education on consciousness. Once again, if there is no understanding about the functioning of consciousness, it will be like working in the dark. When you walk across a dark room and stumble on a table you have to touch it and determine what it is to be able to take your next step. That is why we have to create hypotheses and statistically analyze data. You formulate your hypothesis, or best guess of what you think the reality is, collect data and either accept or reject it based upon that evidence.

Consciousness should be the first thing that any medical practitioner should be trained in. Both Chinese and Indian medicine is rooted in consciousness because without it, would almost be impossible to give great details on all the energy channels and organ systems function and impact on the body. The ancient doctors could move their consciousness inside their own bodies and bring it to specific organs to get information on how they function or their state of imbalance. One can only imagine what medical scientists could do today with all the technology they have if they also started to teach and focus on consciousness.

Consciousness is the energy or undisturbed intelligence that flows through the body at all times.

When we are silent and relaxed, we feel it in the form of rest. It is the same intelligence that rejuvenates us during the night, knows when there is pain in any part of the body, or responds to any threat that you might encounter. It is the energy that we breathe in through the air, which our body assimilates and processes. When you go into a deep state of relaxation or "meditation" you will get a sense of being submerged in it, like you are standing in a swimming pool completely covered in water.

Once you have this experience, you will know your source. Then your whole perception of body will change from a chaotic, random process to one of rhythm and continuum. In that moment, you will also recognize the intricate details of how a human body functions in real time.

Reference of Health

With a lack of understanding of body/mind/consciousness, we have no frame of reference (health) to keep it in balance (disease-free). Since we don't know what balance (healthy state) is, we will not be able to detect or treat it when it starts to slide into an imbalanced state. It is like when you drive your car—you have a sense of balance on the road; you don't go all the way into a ditch before you make a correction.

If you trip on an object and fall, you don't just stay there forever. You pick yourself up and continue to walk again. You can do this because you know how to stand and you have a sense of balance. If you did not know what it meant to be walking upright, you would still be there on the floor. You know balance well enough that if you move away from it; you know how to come back to it.

What is Body Balance?

Ayurveda is a system of understanding that has been around for thousands of years. Ayurveda is made up of two words; "ayur" means life, and "veda" means knowledge or understanding. The first step or foundation of ayurveda is based on the relationship between the body and consciousness. To drive a car, you need to have a car and a driver—your body can be thought of as a car and your consciousness as its driver. How well the car drives depends upon how conscious the driver is. If the driver is asleep, the car

will go nowhere. Without consciousness, your body is just a mechanical device kept going by unknown forces working strictly on mechanical and physical principles. In ayurveda, the body is the periphery and the consciousness is its center—you cannot think of one without the other.

According to ayurveda your body is made up of five elements: earth, water, fire, air and ether. These elements combine in different proportions to fulfill the required functions in the body. An imbalance or diseased state happens when the required elements cannot combine or are disturbed. Understanding and bringing these elements into a balance will bring health and vitality to the body. The three principal methods to bring about this balance are exercises, food choices and element-balancing herbs.

Three basic principles

The body functions with three basic principles: water, fire and air.

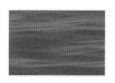 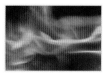 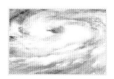

The earth and water elements combine and create the water principle know as kapha—the anabolic principle in your body. The qualities of kapha are: slow, slimy, cool, heavy, liquid, dense, soft and cloudy. In your body the kapha principle, the water and earth elements, stick together and form dense masses such as bones, cartilage, lubrication for the joints, organs, muscles, viscous cellular liquid, and memory liquid (tarpaka kapha in the synaptic clefts, which we discussed in Chapter 5).

The water and fire elements combine and produce pitta—the metabolic principle. This principle functions in the body as hot, sharp, liquid, light, and minor oiliness. The main pitta in your body comes from your stomach and is known as jatara agni (stomach fire) due to all the digestive acid and enzymes. All the enzymes and amino acids that are used in the body for any transformation such as digestion, sensation, and perception are due to the pitta principle in the body. The pitta organs in the body are the intestines, stomach, liver, skin, eyes, blood, and gray matter of the brain. The organs such as the intestines, stomach and liver/gallbladder/spleen are pitta organs because they produce digestive enzymes (pitta elements). The pupil of the eye and the skin are also pitta because they have the fire that is required to transform any impulse into a sensation.

The fire and air elements come together and produce the air principle or vata—the catabolic principle. The qualities of the vata principle that you can use to identify its presence or absence are: dry, light, cold, rough, mobile, subtle, and clear. You can think of them as a tornado. When the time is right, and things need to be moved forward in the body, your body intelligence creates a twister just like nature creates a twister outdoors to move things. When you have a bowel movement during the day, it is the air principle in the colon that is moving the digested food through. If you have a very healthy colon, you will feel a strong movement as the food is pushing through. There are five types of main air principles in the body: prana vayu, udana vayu, samana vayu, apana vayu and vyana vayu.

Prana vayu is the intelligence principle that resides in the center of your brain. When this principle is calm and undisturbed, it reflects as stillness in your life. When this principle is disturbed with thoughts, it becomes either erratic or stagnant. Prana vayu is the principle in your body that performs all the functions. For example, it is the prana vayu that moves into the stomach and directs the digestive process. It acts like a conductor or a manager orchestrating all the required elements to perform the right tasks.

Udana vayu resides between your throat and diaphragm. The breathing and speech processes are caused by udana vayu.

Samana vayu resides in your digestive organs such as your stomach and small intestines. All the movement of the digestive enzymes (through the gall bladder and pancreas) is due to this principle. The pyloric valve is opened and the food is sprayed into the duodenum due to the pressure created by samana vayu under the direction of prana vayu.

Apana vayu resides in your colon and the abdominal area of your body. Removal of feces, urination, and menstrual cycles are governed by this principle.

Vyana vayu is the overall circulatory air principle in the body that governs blood circulation.

When all the three principles function together at their highest level you have optimum health.

Imbalance

If any of the three principles are disturbed, it causes an imbalance in the body known as dosha. The literal translation of the word dosha is "fault" so you can have a fault due to any of the three principles or their combinations going out of balance. The dosha can originate with two possibilities: either too much (vruddhi or to increase) or too little (kshaya, to deplete).

How the principles work together.

When you eat, a lot of processes happen, starting with chewing the food in your mouth. The food gets broken down in your mouth and digestion starts with the secretion of certain enzymes. The food then passes through the esophagus into the stomach. While the food is being broken down in the mouth, a water-based lining is being created in your stomach and esophagus. This lining is essential to protect the stomach wall from the digestive enzymes and hydrochloric acid. The food is then made into a paste by the folds in your stomach. This is done by releasing digestive enzymes and hydrochloric acid and by the folds moving the food to break it down. Once the food is ready and completely homogenized, the air pressure in the stomach (samana vayu) opens the pyloric valve and sprays it into the duodenum.

The creation of the water-based, white lining protecting the stomach and the esophagus is done by the kapha principle. The release of the digestive enzymes and hydrochloric acid is due to the pitta principle and the spraying of the food from the stomach into the duodenum is due to the vata principle. It is very easy to see that if any one of these principles is disturbed, it will cause an imbalance or dosha in the stomach.

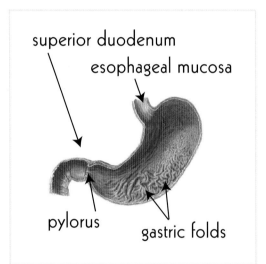

superior duodenum

esophageal mucosa

pylorus

gastric folds

If there is not enough kapha lining in the stomach when you eat your food, you could have gastritis or ulcers in your stomach. If too little hydrochloric acid or enzymes are released due to weak pitta, digestion cannot be completed in the stomach and it will be hard to move the food into the duodenum. This could cause bloating or indigestion, leading to the creation of toxins in the stomach. If too much acid or too many enzymes are being released, this causes burning and ulceration in the stomach. Finally, if there is a weak air principle in the stomach, it will have a hard time opening the pyloric valve causing the food to be pushed back into the esophagus leading to severe heartburn, hiatal hernia or Gastroesophageal Reflux Disease (GERD).

Once the cause of the imbalance is identified, appropriate herbs can be taken. If the imbalance is due to too little kapha lining in the stomach (which causes a burning sensation) it can be brought into a balance with cooling herbs such as Satavari. If not enough acid or enzymes are released for digestion, spices such as black pepper, cumin, or cardamom will bring digestion back into balance. If the cause is due to low air principle and the air is stagnant within the stomach, the ayurvedic herb Dashmoola will bring the air principle back into balance.

This exercise of breaking down a principle, organ or part of a body by each element helps in diagnosing the exact cause of the imbalance. Once the diagnosis is done correctly, powerful herbs, exercises and foods will bring the body back into a state of balance. If you have any ailment in your body, think about all three principles and how they may be impacted. For an in-depth understanding on how to practice the ayurvedic system of body balancing, please see the bibliography for references.

Diagnosis, Diagnosis, Diagnosis

It cannot be overstated. The correct diagnosis of the imbalance is absolutely key in ayurveda. Otherwise, you will not see much improvement in your condition. Spend some time making sure that you have diagnosed the imbalance correctly or at least narrowed it down to one or two options. Then take corrective action via choices of herbs, avoiding or taking certain foods and doing or not doing certain exercises. If your diagnosis is correct, you should see a huge improvement in your condition within 48 to 72 hours. If your condition does not change within 48 hours, just note that your diagnosis was not accurate. Go back to the drawing board again and look at the symptoms thoroughly. How close you are to your body will help you understand these principles and their interactions correctly.

Examples of diagnosis:

If you have a burning sensation, pain with burning sensation, redness, sore or inflamed skin or organs, your pitta principle is probably out of balance. This can be due to the fact that either the kapha (water) and vata (air) principles are at a lower than optimal level or the pitta (fire) principle is at a higher than optimal level. For example, you can have arthritis due to an imbalance in any one of the principles. Therefore there are three types of arthritis—vata, pitta or kapha.

Your lifestyle, food and exercise habits can also cause imbalances in your system. If you are a lean person who runs or jogs a lot on a regular basis, you might have difficulty moving your bowels. This is because your vata and kapha principles are low and your pitta is high in your colon. Low vata and kapha means that there is not enough lubrication and energy to pass the food through. This causes the toxins to accumulate in the colon where they affect bone and tissue creation, giving rise to stiffness and pain-like symptoms. In many cases, toxins will deposit uric acid crystals in the form of pins and needles into the joints. These pins and needles will then tear off parts of the cartilage in the joints of your knees, fingers and feet and cause excruciating pain. This is because you have lost the kapha properties (water lubrication) in the cartilage making it relatively dry. There is no cushion left between the bones anymore and the pins between the joints prick through the bones as you apply pressure on them. To add to this problem, if your foundation or structure is incorrect while you are running, unbalanced pressure will make things worse. So you may think that by running you will reduce weight and look lean and healthy, but there might be other imbalances that you may not see immediately.

In ayurveda, a rule of thumb is to exercise up to 50% of your energy level. This is because your body will need the rest (50%) to fulfill other functions. That is why yoga, Qi-gong exercises, swimming, walking and jogging on soft surfaces are the recommended forms of exercise. If you wish to play competitive sports and avoid short and long-term injuries, do an hour's worth of stretching, relaxation and energy movement exercises before you play. Be mindful of keeping a balance between the three principles and don't just focus on how lean and muscular your body looks in the mirror. If you are playing any sports do the six foundation-building exercises to make sure your posture and body alignment is correct.

If you are a woman you may have gone through a problem with your periods at one time or another. Problems with periods can be due to all three types of imbalances (dosha): vata, pitta and kapha.

Having the vata type of imbalance would mean that you have a low vata or (air principle) in your abdominal area. You will be spotting, feel bloated, have cramps, lower back and abdominal pain and have difficulty starting your period. It is like having a fan that does not work during the middle of the summer. It will get hot and unbearable.

If your pitta is imbalanced (or high) it will, cause inflammation, irritation and stagnation in your period. With too much fire principle pitta where it shouldn't be, your body will become very sensitive—your breasts will be swollen, you might have a burning sensation when passing urine, feel bloated and highly emotional. Then when your period does start, it will be very heavy.

In a kapha imbalance, you will feel bloated and heavy—a classic sign of kapha principle. You might feel congestion and have difficulty starting your period. You will also have a white discharge with your period.

In General
If you feel a sense of constipation, dryness, cold you should look into the imbalances due to the vata (air) principle.

If you see redness, heat, inflammation, sharp pain or burning sensations it is very likely your pitta principle is out of balance.

Imbalances in your body such as a sense of bloating, oily white or yellow discharge and congestion are indications of kapha imbalance. However, this is by no means an exhaustive list of symptoms.

Balancing techniques
Once you know which principle is out of balance, you have two paths to take: If you discover that one of the principles is less than what it should be, then take herbs and do exercises that will enhance that principle and/or reduce the other two principles. If a particular principle is more than what it should be, reducing that particular principle would be your course of action. This can be achieved by taking herbs that reduce it, eating foods that will pacify it, avoiding foods that will aggravate it, and doing the exercises that will bring it into balance. There are situations where you might encounter two or more principles working together; in which case, bringing the two principles into balance and reducing the

third principle would be the course of action. For more information on herbs and foods please refer to the bibliography.

Stress and Digestion

How you chew your food is a good example of how a small thing can impact your body in a big way. Say you eat an apple in a preoccupied way. You chew the apple three times and gulp it down. Chewing is the beginning of a long digestive process. If the first step is incorrect, you can imagine what will happen in the rest of the steps. When you chew, the large food particles are broken down into smaller particles. The enzymes in your saliva such as pancreatic amylase further break down and digest the food at the molecular level. If the first step is not done correctly then it will certainly put more stress on the rest of the digestive processes.

When the half-chewed food reaches the stomach, it will lack several enzymes that never arrived in the required quantities. Now we have a problem. The stomach cannot do its job in breaking the food down. In despair, it just pushes the undigested food over to your duodenum. Your congested liver is not producing the optimal level of bile and the story is the same with your pancreas. The stomach, duodenum and intestines have lost their tone because you couldn't exercise or were too busy with other things.

These organs cannot collect all the processed food and send it to the liver in an efficient manner. The rest of the body is going to be starved for nutrients. When this happens you feel weak and have less energy. Since you feel weak, you eat more highly-processed foods because you feel you need energy immediately. In addition, your Type B thoughts are keeping you totally stressed and sleep-deprived. You find yourself gaining weight. As you gain weight, you start to feel weak because you are moving less. You need a break and you find yourself tired all the time. The weight keeps adding on and it is hard to take it off. This downward spiral may be why 65% of Americans are overweight, of which 33% are obese.

I have watched many people eating, and my conclusion is that at least 95% don't chew their food more than three times. By doing this, they will never actually taste the food and could also develop eating disorders.

We don't chew our food and unfortunately there are no teeth in our stomach that can correct this problem. In the West, the obesity problem reigns because of lack of chewing. Chewing not only breaks down the food, but also gives a sense of taste. One of the ways we come to know things as they are is through taste. When this faculty is deprived, our innate nature craves it. This is how food cravings are developed— because we are not able to satisfy our sense of taste. The problem happens when we eat food just for the taste, but our consciousness is so disturbed by both outside and inside stimulus that we are unable to notice what we are eating. We then have to eat large quantities just to get a small glimpse of the taste in our consciousness. This is how overeating and food addiction happen. When we eat consciously, in a relaxed way, enjoying the taste, our bodies process the food efficiently and its essence nourishes us.

The Six Steps of Digestion

Let's take a journey into the body and see what is really happening. The best way to visit is through your mouth. Imagine that you are eating a piece of apple with awareness and alertness. You are conscious through the entire chewing process. Your mouth is the first place where the food is chopped up and mixed with digestive enzymes that break down the carbohydrates. Six salivary glands open from the sides of the cheeks and secrete saliva, since the oral cavity needs to be constantly lubricated. Chewing is a very important part of the digestive principle.

Through taste, the tongue gives the whole body information about what needs to be done with the food. Six tastes can be felt on the tongue: sweet, sour, salty, pungent, bitter and astringent. Each taste will impact different parts of the body. Excess sweets will impact the pancreas. Foods high in salt will make the body hold more water resulting in the high blood pressure of those who are already hypertensive.

As the food moves through the digestive organs in the body, it also goes through a transformation in taste: In the mouth it is sweet, in the stomach it is sour, in the duodenum it is salty, in the jejunum it is bitter, in the ileum (small intestine) it is pungent and finally in the colon it is astringent. Part of ayurvedic diagnosis and treatment is based upon which stage of digestion is impacted or out of balance.

The broken-down apple mixed with saliva and enzymes moves through the esophagus and ends up in the stomach (the kitchen stove). You need two things, water and fire, to cook or digest the food. The upper part of the stomach included in the gastrointestinal tract starts to secrete a mucous-like membrane that is liquid, soft and oily. This water element helps distribute the heat evenly throughout the food.

Food Enters
Liver
Stomach
Spleen
Duodenum
Pancreas
Ascending colon
Descending colon
Cecum
Ileum

Hydrochloric acid acts as the fire element by raising the heat and breaking down the food further into smaller pieces. The hormone gastrin causes the release of pepsin, an enzyme that aids in the digestion of proteins. Due to the release of all the enzymes and the acids, the taste of the food in your stomach is sour. Once the food is digested in the stomach, it moves to the duodenum through the opening of the pyloric valve.

Here, the food is mixed with the bile secreted by the liver through the gallbladder and pancreatic enzymes: amylase, lipase and trypsin. The food that arrives from the stomach is acidic and the bile and pancreatic enzymes are alkaline in nature. When acid foods meet with the alkaline enzymes, they turn the food into salt and water. This aids in the breaking down of fats and proteins.

The salty food then moves into the jejunum, which is a part of the small intestines. This place can be thought of as kitchen oven or the stove where the food will be cooked (digested). The enzymes in the jejunum have a pungent taste with hot and sharp qualities. The hot qualities will cause the absorption of food essence.

From the jejunum, the pungent, processed food moves into the ileum, the longest part of the small intestines. Due to the presence of bile and other enzymes in this part of the small intestine, the food has a bitter taste. In the entire intestines from jejunum through the ileum, the function is absorption of the nutrients (essence). This can be seen in the network of veins that are connected from the small intestines to the liver.

Through the ileocecal valve, the food enters into the cecum. Now, the food has an astringent taste which has a dry feeling. Astringent taste is what you feel after you eat a lot of corn (like a cotton mouth). When the processed food arrives into the colon, it starts to get dry and ready to be pushed out of the body. In the colon, the body is trying to get all the nutrients out of the food before it is eliminated. That is the reason why it is important to eat vegetables and greens because they are soft and can hold

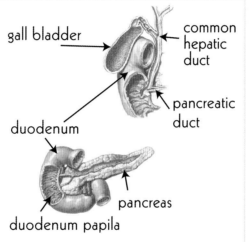

gall bladder

common hepatic duct

duodenum

pancreatic duct

pancreas

duodenum papila

water, helping the digested food move through the colon.

Importance of Consciousness

For your body to remain free from disease and stress it is necessary for your consciousness to remain undisturbed at all times. This should be the only goal in your life. If this goal is missed, no other goals will be achieved.

If you are the owner/manager of a store with six employees, you have to give them clear directions. If you don't give any directions, and you are hardly at the store, how long do you think you will be in business? In your absence, some employees will come and some won't. Things will go missing. This is exactly how we manage our bodies. Since you are not conscious, with all the energy consumed in your Type B thoughts, there is no one available to give any directions. So your stomach may do its function, or it may not. If it does not, it doesn't care because the consciousness/manager is not present. All the work piles up on the liver. It never gets a break, but you are not aware of that, so it gets clogged, diseased and stressed. There is total chaos. Somehow or the other, you manage your life with pills, inhalers and shots. Your body becomes like a black box where food enters one end and comes out the other. You don't know how or why. Until one day things get so bad that nothing can be done. You meet your fate.

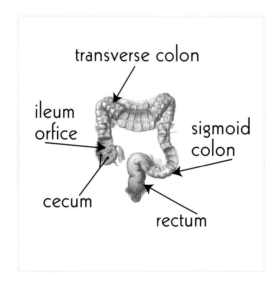

Managing Expectations and Comparisons

Start to look at your body in light of the three principles: vata, pitta and kapha. If you have an ailment that has been bothering you, or know of a friend or family member who has an ailment, then break their symptoms down by these three principles. Look at their history, what type of body they have, what they generally eat, their sleep and exercise patterns, their family history, etc.

Create a good understanding of their situation and narrow their symptoms down to one or two imbalances in the principles. Read more on the subject with the books listed in the bibliography. Find the herbs that will balance the ailment you are studying. Find out why the herb or mixture of herbs that you have found is the best solution. Read up on the herbs

themselves and find out where they grow and if there are side effects to taking them. What is the correct dosage of the herb for the ailment?

In addition, read the next chapter thoroughly and see what exercises would work the best based upon your diagnosis of the ailment. Do your exercises every day without expectations. Let your consciousness and your body be balanced each and every day and you will remain disease free, full of energy and conscious all the time.

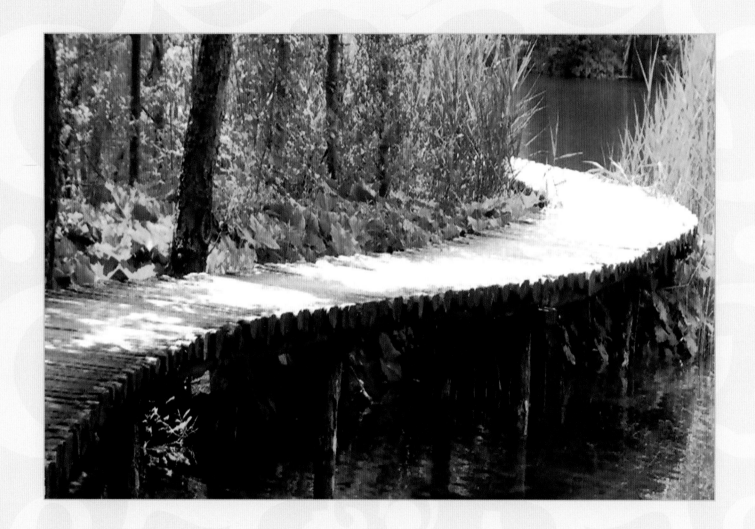

Yoga (Reunion)

योगः चित्तवृत्तिनिर्धः

In Yoga all disturbances to the consciousness ceases.

What is Yoga:

संयोगे योग इत्युक्तो जीवात्मपरमात्मनोः

Yoga is the re-union of living self with the Supreme Self (Yajnavalkya)
the highest, pure infinite knowledge of consciousness is attained.

सर्वचिन्ता परित्यागो निश्चिन्तो योग उच्यते :

To silence the mind leaving all mental activity is yoga (Yoga Shâstra).

पुरुषस्यात्यन्तिकस्वरूपावस्थितिहेतुः चित्तवृत्तिनिरोधो योगः

The silencing of the mind's activities which leads to the complete realization of the intrinsic
nature of the Supreme Person is called yoga (Yoga Sâra Sangraha, p.1 Adyar ed).

What is an Asana (Posture)

स्थिरसुखमासनम्

To remain motionless for a long time without effort is an Asana
(Patanjali, Yoga Darshana 2, 46).

पयत्नशैथिल्यानन्तसमापत्तिभ्याम्

The aim of the bodily postures is secured when the physical reactions of the body are
eliminated and mind dissolves into the infinite (Patanjali, Yoga Darshana 2, 47).

This section is dedicated to Gurudev B.K.S. Iyengar

Say you are taking a walk in the park and you come across a small stream. You want to cross the stream and you find an old, dead tree trunk, well-placed by Nature, that connects one side to the other. Given your situation, you clearly know what to do, but you have to come up with things that you know will help you cross. This is not something that you do every day, but within yourself, you start to put things together. You ascertain the situation: how deep is the water, how sturdy and stable is the tree trunk, is it wet with algae or dry and what is the distance you are trying to cover. Once you feel very confident, you place your first foot carefully on the wood, and when you have more confidence, both your feet get on the trunk.

Wow! You didn't think of alertness and balance before, and all of a sudden they become very important. You find that extending your arms gives you the balance that you need to keep steady on the tree trunk. It is your alertness and balance that is going to help you cross this stream. Once you have the balance and are not in a rush, you find that you are in the moment, and the walk seems easy. Eventually, you cross over to the other side feeling a sense of exhilaration, happiness and accomplishment. Crossing the stream becomes a device for your transformation.

What you have just experienced is the state of yoga where you saw and connected what was in front of you. Once you connected, you knew exactly what to do even though nobody was prompting you or leading you through the walk. The understanding and connection with the environment is yoga, and all the adjustments that your body made are the exercises or asanas.

Everything that we do in our lives can be divided into two parts: the intelligence or the consciousness and the act or the physical process itself. When these two parts are disconnected or absent, there is chaos. The disconnection occurs when unrelated chatter distracts you from whatever you are doing. On the other hand, when the two components come together in balance, we have evolution and transformation.

All the tools presented in the previous nine chapters will help you remain chatter-free, letting your undivided consciousness flow into everything that you do. This understanding is central to the Oriental understanding of life, and is the foundation of ayurveda, yoga and Qi-gong. In ayurveda, the consciousness is called "purush" (masculine energy, Yin, center) and creativity is called "prakruthi" (feminine energy, Yang, the periphery). The Chinese and Indian terminology may seem opposite but they are not because yin is the feminine energy which the Indian system identifies as the center or the masculine energy. They both are looking at two different characteristics of the same phenomenon. To keep this

Wherever the consciousness is at its highest the ego is at its lowest and vice/versa.

understanding clear, think of a bicycle wheel. A bicycle wheel has two components: the center and the periphery or the wheel itself. You cannot have a functional wheel with only one component—you will always need both together.

Say, for example, you come home in a hurry and leave your car keys some place where you normally don't put them. The next time you need the keys, you will have to look all over your house to find them. If you are in a hurry, you may feel unnecessary stress. In this case, the act and consciousness got disconnected which lead to chaos. This makes it clear how important consciousness (or the center) is when doing anything. Unfortunately, in our lives, we never got trained in the most important thing—bringing consciousness to everything that we do, so we go from one thing to the next almost blindly.

Another definition of yoga is: a state where all acts are done with consciousness. The practice of yoga asanas is a deliberate process of learning to bring the act and consciousness together. The understanding is that once this learning goes deep within you, it will manifest into other things of your life.

Asanas and Yoga

Your yoga practice should be like driving your car or riding a bicycle, where all your movement and adjustments come from what is in front of you. When you drive a car, your eyes are on the road and you are conscious of everything in front of and around you. All the adjustments that you make to your car are made based on what you see and feel. Your legs or hands don't make the decision on their own; they are merely tools for your consciousness, which sees everything. Your practice should be one where your consciousness is what gives you the next direction or move and makes all the subtle required adjustments. Then there is no question of having an accident, or getting hurt, or comparing your form or stretch with others.

A Mother Crocodile

I saw a show on TV about a 20-foot long crocodile mother who had just delivered over 20 eggs. The mother croc had to move the eggs to a place where they could hatch undisturbed. She lifted up each egg with her mouth, in between her teeth so gently that not one egg was disturbed or broken, and dropped the egg in the pouch of her mouth. She patiently did this process for all of the eggs and gently moved quite some distance where she dug a hole with her fore and hind limbs and deposited each one, still without disturbing any of them. This to me is the definition of yoga—being totally connected—where each cell or pore of your being is soaked with consciousness. If you are a human, in that moment your mind will have totally disappeared. There is no way a thought can enter and you merge into the infinite.

Our body is made of five elements: earth, water, fire, air and ether. It will be beneficial for you to understand the elements, their impact on your body, when they are in balance or out of balance and finally what you can do to keep them in balance. In short, you are trying to understand the environment of your body/mind/consciousness. The yoga asanas and the Qi-gong movements will bring a balance to the elements in your body. There are no expectations on the outcome; you are interested in fulfilling your part in the process of regaining your health and vitality.

The asanas are laid out on the basis of which elements they balance or bring forth and are listed as follows:

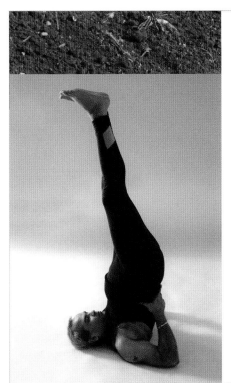

Earth (prithvi) or Grounding happens when you bring your head to the earth, or your mouth opens into the earth like a tree that has its mouth (roots) in the earth. When your head touches the earth, the consciousness within you connects with the universal consciousness all around you.

The point from where the consciousness leaves your body is called "Bramarindra" or "Gu-Shen." If you are silent and undisturbed, you will feel a tingling sensation in the soles of your feet while it will feel like your head is buried into the earth and a deep relaxation will come over you.

All yoga positions where your head touches the earth will balance the earth element in your body.

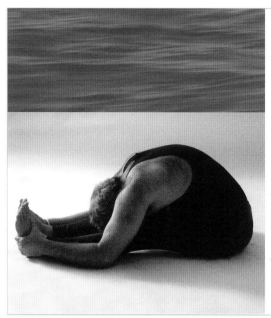

The Water element (panni) is brought into balance with all forward bends. In a forward bend, a lot of pressure is exerted upon your digestive organs. The pancreas, as per ayurveda, is the water organ. In addition, over 90% of your serotonin is produced in your abdominal area. It is your serotonin that gives you that high, positive, relaxed feeling. When pressure is applied to this region of the body and you are silent enough to sense it, you will find your whole body has turned into water. Your chatter will dissolve quickly in forward bends and your whole body will become extremely flexible.

All yoga positions where your head comes to your knees and pressure is applied to your abdominal area will balance the water element.

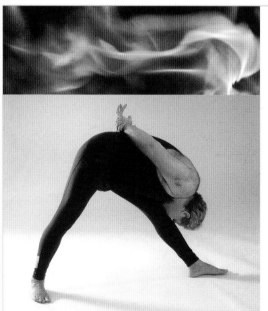

Fire (aagh) constitutes all the metabolic principles in your body. Any type of digestive processing in your body is due to this element. Fire breaks down things into two parts, one that will be used immediately and one that will be used by the next process. For example, the fire from hydrochloric acid breaks the food down to be used by the stomach and by the small intestines where further absorption will happen.

All the standing positions will balance the fire element in your body. The key is the soles of your feet. When you are silent and your body is grounded, you will feel a certain heat in the soles of your feet and feel a sensation of fire coming out from them. The Chinese masters call this phenomenon "the bubbling well." In these standing positions your whole body will feel the heat. If done right, this will transform into your tejas (body intelligence).

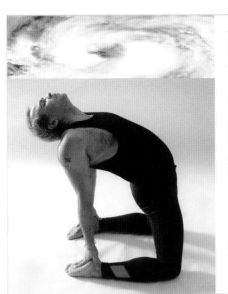

Air (vayu) is the catabolic or the movement principle in your body. All things that move in your body are moved by the air principle. For example, the circulation of blood through your body is due to Vyana vayu.

More people are affected by the air principle than any other, because it is the most subtle of all. If this principle is disturbed it impacts several other principles in your body. For example, when you have constipation, you could have a weak air principle in your colon. If left unchecked, it will lead to several problems both short term (breathing congestion and headaches) and long-term (all types of arthritis).

All back bends will help bring this principle into balance. When you are silent and do back bends, you will feel a sense of cool dryness all over your body. Dryness is a classic sign of the vayu principle

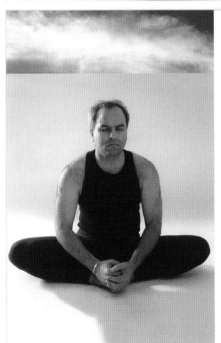

Ether (aakash) is pure, undisturbed consciousness or the state of yoga itself. This is the purush or the center of the wheel, a state of pure conscious alertness. Nothing in your life should happen without this element, especially when doing your exercise practice. Doing anything without this element is like driving your car with your eyes shut. When you can see clearly what lies in front of you, it takes away all the fears, desires and other virtual realities from your consciousness. When you drive your car completely consciously, you don't fear anything. However, that will not be the case when your eyes are closed—you will be understandably paranoid.

This is the one that creates all the balance in your life. It brings a certain quality to whatever you do like driving your car or cleaning your house.

When you open the doors and windows of your house, taking away all the barriers, the outside air moves into your house and merges with the inside air. In the same way, when all the doors and windows of your body are open without any disturbance, the universal consciousness naturally flows into your body. It mingles and merges with what is trapped within your body and lets it flow. This is how you bring this element into balance.

Yoga and Qi-gong

The Qi-gong exercises work on a different principle than yoga; all the elements are brought together and balanced at the same time. The Qi-gong exercises balance the three centers in the front of the body by moving the energy from the brain to the stomach (first dan-tian to the third dan-tian). In the yoga system, the energy is moved from the lower spine to the top of the head. Both systems are complementary. Qi-gong exercises are yoga in motion and asanas are yoga in stillness or postures.

Qi-gong exercises are harder to do because they require 100% of the ether element up front, meaning no disturbance at all. In other words, you have to be silent to experience anything. If you become silent, they will do wonders. When you are silent, it does not matter how your arms or legs move because you are not moving them, they are being moved by the universal consciousness (Heaven Qi). It is like a piece of wood that is flowing with the river. The piece of wood does not direct the river, the river directs the wood whichever way it likes. In fact, the piece of wood and the river become one.

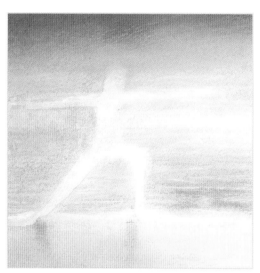
Disappearnce of body into consciousness

The best way to know the state of yoga is through the Qi-gong exercises. These are slow-moving, gentle, yet extremely powerful exercises bringing your energy up to the center of your brain—see chapter 3. Once you are in the state of oneness, move from one exercise (stretch) to the next and stay in it as long as you can. Don't concern yourself about coming out or how long to stay in each position. The beauty of yoga exercises is that each exercise works on your entire body and not just one small part. Each asana is complete in itself.

Many Situations

When we think of balance, we are unconsciously thinking of a center—whatever that may be. For example, while walking in the park, you accidentally hit a stone and your body lunges forward and you fall. You will say you lost your balance or your body was unable to center. Yoga works on the principle of being in your center and consciously knowing what happens when you move away from it. In yoga, your body is the medium and your consciousness is the silent director.

The yoga asanas can be thought of as many situations that we purposefully put our body in to know what happens. Each situation gives us a new piece of information about ourselves at all levels (body/mind/consciousness). If you put yourself in different positions and are conscious, you will be able to tell if you are centered or off-center in the position. The beauty is that as soon as you realize that you are off-center in any position, your consciousness starts to bring your back into the center. This is yoga where all that needs to happen is awareness; beyond that, no effort is necessary as the corrective process begins on its own.

Breathing (Pranayama):

This topic is the center of many yoga and Qi-gong practices in the world. Breathing is a subtle relationship between your body and the universal consciousness. It is a well-known fact that your breath and the state of your mind are related. If your mind is calm your breathing will be deep and vice/versa. All the breathing techniques are designed with the argument that if the breath is altered then the functioning of the mind can be altered as well. So the breath is like a controller of the mind. Since we don't know how to control the mind, we can control the breath, which in turn will control the mind.

An important connection is made here. However, there is one problem with this thinking—it is only temporary. Let us say that you are sitting in silence and focusing on your breath and suddenly a thought comes into your head and you get engaged. You now have two processes going on: your practice of breathing and your internal discussion with the thought. This division in your consciousness causes you to become unaware of the breath, which is lost in the unconscious because the internal talk has taken over. Your thoughts are based on your expectations, comparisons and virtual realities of things, and they are so rooted in you that unless you deal with them directly nothing will work. Calming yourself down with breath alone is like trying to calm or control a big African elephant by its tail—it is going to be rough, if not impossible.

When you are trying to calm your mind with the breath, in essence you are trying to calm your expectations and comparisons. While you may be successful at times in pacifying your mind with the breathing exercises, you will find that as soon as you are in the real world all your expectations and comparisons are back. This is the greatest frustration. So what does one do? You cannot just give up the world and move into a monastery, because your expectations and comparisons will follow you there. Actually, they may get worse, because now you have left the real world's distractions. The best thing to do is to deal with your expectations and comparisons directly and not through some unclear surrogates.

Breathing with No Expectation

Try this now if you can. Sit or lie down in silence and let the breath come and leave your body as it wants. Feel like you have opened the doors and windows of your house and the air is flowing through as it wants. There is no effort on your part to make anything happen. While the breath is moving in and out have no expectations of it. Whatever way your breath moves, you have no expectations of it. Let your awareness be with the breath, but with no expectations. If you are successful in not having any expectations you will find that you will come into a state of oneness.

If you stayed with the breath with no expectations, you may discover that you are clearly feeling a pressure point about 1 to 1.5 inches below your navel. This is your hara center or third dan-tian. Once you start to feel this center, you have taken the first step towards your transformation. If you continue to practice this technique on a daily basis, along with other movements and exercises as shown, this center will clearly become your home and you will be constantly aware of it.

Sage Patanjali Says

In the Yoga Sutra 2, 51: बाह्याभ्यन्तर विषय आक्षेपी चतुर्थः Bahya abhyantara vishaya akshepi caturthah

The fourth type of pranayama transcends the external and internal pranayamas, which is effortless and non-deliberate.

This pranayama or breathing can only be compared to breathing in a mother's womb. The child in the womb has no breathing of its own; whenever the mother breathes, the child breathes. You will feel like you are being breathed and someone is bringing the breath to you. It will give you a feeling that someone wants you to be here and you are very much part of this existence.

When the energy moves into the center of the brain, the breathing will almost stop, but you will feel a sense of total wakefulness. Your consciousness will be undisturbed, and for the first time, you will also realize that it could not be disturbed even if you wanted. The distance between your mind and consciousness will be the same as the distance between the earth and sky. You will also realize that your mind was nothing but impressions made on the consciousness—like when you shine a flashlight on the wall. Shining the flashlight does not change or alter the wall. Once you see this experience clearly within yourself, your mind will lose its grip on you. You will be awakened from your unconscious sleep.

No Expectations and Asana Practice

You must be wondering how having no expectations during your yoga asana or natural breathing practice will help them? Or what is the connection between no-expectation, yoga asana and breath? Whenever you are doing anything, your mind automatically places a picture of your expectation in your brain (more specifically, between your eyebrows). That is why many times, even before trying, you may say or must have heard people say to you: "I cannot do that" or "It looks like it will hurt my back" or "I don't think I will benefit from the experience." What you are narrating is this picture that has been placed in your mind. This picture is the expectation of what will happen to you by going through the act.

For example, while doing the stretch shown, before you know it an image will be placed in your mind. Once the picture is in place, you will follow the picture and not the body. The comparison process in your mind will compare your stretching to the picture and not to your body. This will cause you to over-extend, strain or not do much at all depending on your picture. Have you noticed people in the gym who look at their bodies trying to match their physical selves with the pictures in their minds of themselves? The entire aim of yoga is to erase these mind-pictures, and the process of placing any picture in your mind in the future. This is freedom. Freedom from the process of your mind that floods you with old information even before you have tried the new action, and robs you of your own experience — freedom from constant analysis of the pictures in your brain. Your aches, pain and stiffness also come from these pictures or expectations. You must have heard people say, "I am getting old and having walking problems because they are a part of becoming old." and similar arguments based on age, gender, or income disposition. These types of arguments are nothing but your expectations or pictures placed within you.

Breaking this process can happen when you say that you don't need a picture to do this or any other act. When you go into a posture with no expectations, you essentially erase the picture, which releases the energy tied into the picture, and all your energy flows right into the posture. This is why kids can do things easily, gracefully and full of innocence, because the picture process is not yet formed in them.

Things to remember:
While doing the asanas and the movements, have no expectations. Let the body move in and out of asanas (stretches) and Qi-gong movements

without desiring anything from it. No expectations while being in the movement or stretch will transform an ordinary movement into divinity.

In all the exercises, feel like you are sitting in water. Why water? We all live in the source of our energy. For us it is the air we breathe; if we did not have air we would be dead in less than three minutes. For all living beings in the sea, it is the water itself. You can imagine how a fish fights for life when removed from its source. "God" or existence is all around you and you live in it. When we breathe, we breathe in god and the same happens when we breathe out. Did you know that you breathe through your skin as well? If all the pores in your body were shut by some means and only your nostrils were left open, you would start to suffocate. Breathing is happening without you even knowing about it. When you totally relax and connect with this source, your pores will dilate and let the life energy come into the body like wind moving through an open window. As you connect with the life source you will become it. In fact, when you totally relax into your movements you will feel like you are moving in water. This is the easiest way to connect with existence or universal consciousness.

When doing the yoga stretches, at times you might feel some pain or discomfort. This is your body complaining as you try to change it. Perhaps certain muscles, tendons, ligaments or cartilage have not moved for some time. When your consciousness guides the movement, it will know exactly what to do. The consciousness will relax and dilate (open and loosen) your body and you will encounter less pain. It is like when you are trying to start an old piece of equipment. You have to do several things to get it up and running. This is exactly what you are going to encounter. Just remember—no expectations and no comparisons.

Your asana and movement practice is not a one-day-a-week affair. Imagine if you took a course at a university and you never opened your books or did your assignments. What type of understanding of the subject would you have? If you do your stretches and movements one or two days a week, it will further stiffen your body and you will not see much flexibility and very likely drop out from the practice. It would be like you made it to the door of a beautiful palace and then turned back without entering.

If you are totally relaxed when doing the exercises, your eyes might roll up and point between the eyebrows. Do not panic! This is exactly what should happen. The rolling of your eyes is an indication that the energy is moving into the center of the brain. In addition, the tip of your tongue might touch the soft palate in the top of your mouth.

In the beginning, do only those stretches that you can do easily without hurting or straining yourself. You are not training for any competition or medal. You can do all the Qi-gong exercises without any problem even if you are in a wheelchair.

You can do all the asanas starting with earth and ending with ether or vice versa.

For the first few times you can keep your eyes open, but after that, do all the asanas and movements with your eyes closed. With your eyes open your energy moves out and will have a harder time reaching the center of your brain. Also, you will be able to feel things better if your eyes are closed because the energy will flow into feeling things rather than seeing and analyzing.

A yoga mat and yoga blocks are two very good investments. A yoga mat is to a yoga practitioner what a good pair of running shoes is to a runner. The yoga mat should be the non-slippery and washable kind. You can support yourself with yoga blocks that can be bought at any health food store or sporting goods stores.

Mandatory Foundation Exercises

The importance of the foundation exercises explained in the previous chapter cannot be over emphasized. Those six exercises should be done every day without fail if you want to stand upright and walk correctly. In the first experience you have with them, you will find how powerful they are in centering your body. You will be able to stand and walk absolutely straight and center.

I recommend that you buy a new pair of flat shoes and discontinue using your old shoes. For example, if you were putting too much pressure on one side of your foot then your shoes will have that imbalance already worked in. If you put too much pressure on the sides of your shoes, your shoes will be worn out more on the sides then the middle. Similarly, if you walk on your heels then the heels on your shoes will be worn out more than any other part of the sole.

Your exercise routine should have the six mandatory exercises and any other exercise that you wish to do from this chapter. For your convenience, the DVD has the six mandatory exercises incorporated into the rest of the exercises in a routine.

Preparation Exercises for Movements

If you have to transform or reshape a ball of iron into a flat-shaped plate, you will have to melt it first. In the same way, when you are putting your body into so many forms, you will have to melt it enough to be able to move deeply into the forms. Our molten form is the energy body that we are going to transform into.

1) Standing forward bend	2) Back bend	3) Side bend

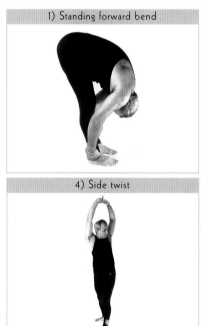 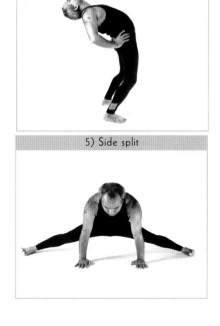 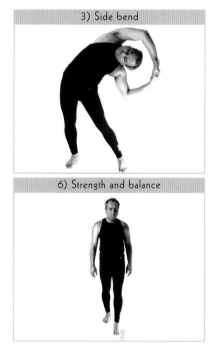

4) Side twist	5) Side split	6) Strength and balance

Becoming aware of your energy body is like opening your eyes before you embark on this journey. Your consciousness will guide you through all of the forms because it will to give you details on each and every aspect of your body. If you let your spirit lead you

through the movements every moment will be transformative and there will be no coming back.

Standing upright, with bare feet (if possible) shoulder-width apart. Keeping your body completely still and totally relaxed, and your eyes open in a soft gaze. Stand in this position for at least ten minutes. If you are silent, undisturbed, and relaxed, you will see your energy rising up to your head. It will make your whole body soft and supple.

Qi-gong Rocker

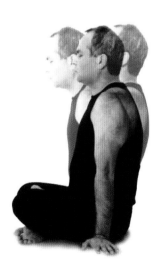

Place your palms on both sides of your hips, slightly bend your elbows and rock your upper body back and forth starting from the lower spine. All your movement should originate from the lower spine. Go slowly like you are moving in water.

This powerful movement will relax you and keep your energy moving upwards to the center of your head.

This movement will balance the energy between your first and third dan-tian.

Qi-gong Head Move

Move your head forward all the way down until your chin touches the groove in the front of your collar bone. Stay there as long as you like and then gently lift your head up and bring it all the way back as far as it can go. Stay there as long as you like. Then bring your head into the center and move to the left and stay as long as possible. Then gently move to the right. Come back to the center only when you are ready. Repeat if your consciousness guides you so.

We store a lot of tension in our head, neck and shoulder area because we use them the most and that's where we hold stress. This exercise will release the energy from your head which will end up in your third dan tian. It will feel like early summer in Alaska where large chunks of ice melt and dissolve into the ocean.

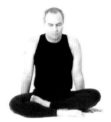 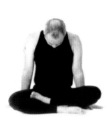 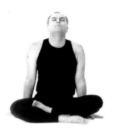 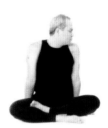 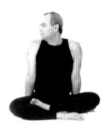

Becoming-One Qi-gong movement

Let your arms move up to shoulder level. Your palms gently move up facing out and pointing upwards. Each move is not done by you, it happens to you—slow and deliberate. Let your arms stay up as long as your consciousness intends. Then slowly, they will start to come down. Let this movement happen to you for at least three to five minutes.

Once again, this movement will move the energy through your body, refreshing it each time. If you are silent, you will feel extremely grounded, like your feet have taken root in the earth.

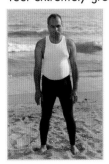 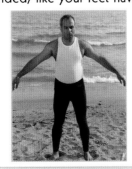 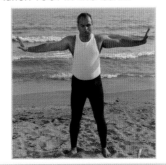 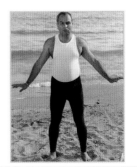 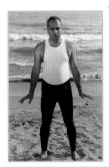

Body Energizing Qi-gong Movement

Move your left or right arm up like some one is moving it for you. Bring it up to shoulder height and move your palm facing forward pointing upwards. Then move your arm down while simultaneously moving the other arm up. Continue this movement for three to four minutes. If you allow this movement to happen, you will find that you are actually swimming in the energy. The energy will be felt so clearly that it will be hard to miss. This exercise will circulate your energy starting from the soles of your feet, moving all the way up, and then bringing it back to the start. All Qi-gong exercises are like taking a spiritual bath.

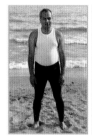 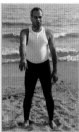 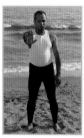 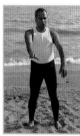 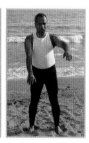 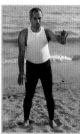 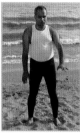 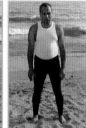

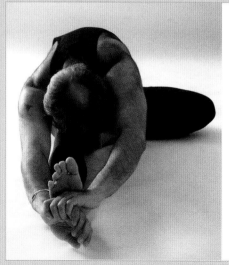

(Head on knees) Janu Sirsasana

Bring your right foot forward and your left foot next to your right thigh. Keep your right knee straight, and let your chin move down to your right knee. Stretch from the lower spine. Totally relax into the posture like you have dissolved into it. Stay in it until your consciousness is ready to move you once again to do the other side.

Initially, you might feel pain in your lower back or your hamstrings. Relax and embrace the pain in those parts. This posture balances your kapha (water principal), tones your internal organs and stretches all the muscles in your legs (especially hamstrings), your lower and upper back.

Managing Expectations and Comparisons

Ah Ha Asana or (Sukha Asana, Blissful Pose)

Simple, yet extremely deep postures are hard to describe because they bring all five elements together more clearly.

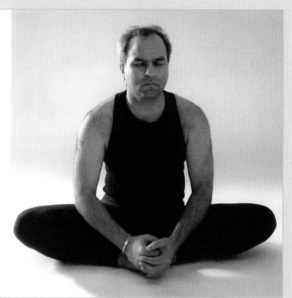

Bring the soles of your feet together and hold them with your palms. Relax your groin, hips, back and let your knees fall to the floor. Once again, this opens the lower spine in a deep way.

This asana can be used as a measure to the level of relaxation or stress in your body. Each time you do your practice come to this posture and stay in it. If your hips are open, groin, arms, legs and shoulders are relaxed, then you know you are headed in the right direction.

Restraint Angle Stretch (Baddha Konasana)

From sukha asana let your consciousness guide you to bring your head forward. Go as far as you can, stop and become blissful. This is a tough exercise if you have not done much stretching before, but we are not in a hurry anyway. Once again, if you let go and relax, you will find that you will go further than you thought. Keep your jaw relaxed.

If there are any thoughts that stray into your consciousness, bring your energy back to the center of your head. If you have a hard time due to chatter then read and follow directions from chapters one to five to eliminate chatter.

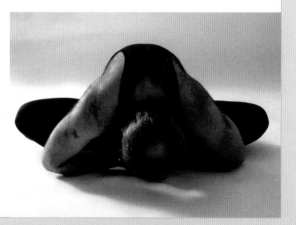

This is a must-do for all females. It will open up all the muscles joining your hip and groin area while opening up the energy block in the base of your spine.

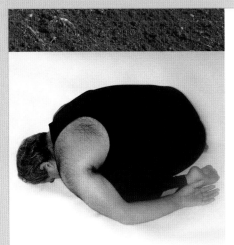

Becoming the Earth (Grounding exercises)
Hero's pose or Child or Fetal pose, Tibetan meditation pose (Virasana)

Bend your legs so that you are sitting on them. Then let the consciousness move your body forward until your head touches the ground. Stay in it until consciousness wants you to move.

It is a position where you will feel relaxed just like when you were in your mother's womb—hence, it is called fetal pose.

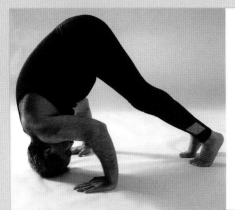

Half-Supported Head Stand (Ardha Salamba Sirsasana I).
Bring your head down to the earth extend your legs back and move your knees away from the floor. If you are worried about your neck and head then keep your knees on the floor. It will work as well.

If you are relaxed while in this position, it will strengthen your head and neck area.

Total Body Posture or Shoulder Stand (Sarvangasana)

Lay down flat on your back and bring both of your legs up by bending at the hips. Then let your legs come over further pushing forward on your lower back with your palms and bringing your lower back away from the floor on to your shoulders. Keep your legs straight up while supporting your lower back with your palms. Your chin should touch the space between the collar bones. If you are silent and relaxed you will feel a sense of warm energy right on the base of your throat (thyroid gland).

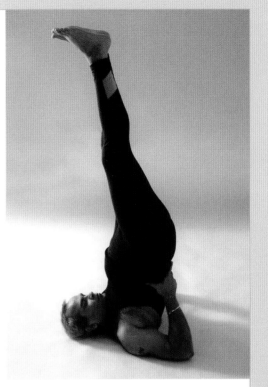

If you don't have enough strength to do this posture, you can do this stretch next to the wall. While squatting on the floor, bring your buttocks next to the edges where the floor and the wall meet. Then kick your legs up against the supporting wall, while you are laying on the floor. At this point, your body should look like a right triangle. Your legs are supported by the wall and your back is flat to the floor.

Next, press your feet against the supporting wall and your bottom will lift away from the floor. Then, bring your palms underneath your lower back to support it. Your knees will be bent at a right angle when you are in this position.

Don't overextend yourself at your neck or you might get a sprain. Make sure you are relaxed while in this position, and at no time should the pressure be on your head or neck. All the pressure should fall only on your shoulders. If you find yourself exerting pressure on your neck or head then gently get out of the posture. Take a blanket fold it to about 1 to 1.5 inches thick and place it underneath your body, from your shoulders down and do the exercise again. The blanket will essentially keep your neck away from the floor which will give you about 1 inch of space when you do the exercise.

There are not enough good things that can be written about this posture. The most important thing is that it brings all the blood to the hypothalamus, pituitary, pineal and thyroid glands. Since it is a grounding position, it will reverse the flow of energy through your legs and out. It is like getting a cosmic shower. It will relax you completely. Stay in it and enjoy the balance as long as your consciousness wants.

Advanced poses

All advanced poses should be done only if you are confident and have practiced the basic poses for at least four to six months. If you are not sure or are not confident then don't attempt them at this time. Your practice with the foundational poses will develop a strong relationship between your consciousness and your body. Then let her (consciousness) guide you through the poses. Remember no expectations and no comparisons.

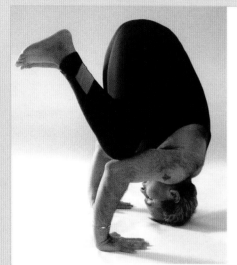

Half Head Stand (Ardha Salamba Sirsasana II)

With your knees bent, sit straight up on your calves. Bring both your palms to the floor on the side in front of you. Make sure that both palms are in a straight line. Place the top of your head in between your palms about a foot forward from your palms. The place where your head touches the floor and the center of your palms will make a symmetrical triangle.

Lift your knees up from the floor and place either your right or left knee on the elbow on the same side. Then bring the other knee on to its elbow as well. Keep a balance between the three points of your two palms and your head.

Keep your eyes closed and body totally relaxed. Enjoy this posture as the first step to a head stand. This is a true fetal position. If you get it right, and are totally relaxed, you will never want to get out of this position.

Once again the blood flows to your brain. The key in all the grounding positions is the weight of the spine. Your lower spine and hip will get some rest as you take away the gravity. You will feel like you are on air and your walk and posture will improve tremendously.

One-Foot Shoulder Stand (Ek Pada Sarvanga Asana)

Doing the shoulder stand correctly and comfortably is a must before attempting this asana.

Extra precaution should be taken to place no pressure on the head and neck.

As described previously, this posture has many benefits such as increasing the blood supply to critical glands. This exercise also tones your colon and will help with elimination process.

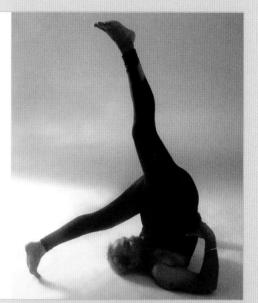

One-Foot Sideways Shoulder Stance (Parasvaika Pada Sarvangasana)

Bring yourself to the shoulder stand, and when you are totally still, let either your left or right foot come down gently to the floor.

Make sure you are not putting any pressure on your neck or head and that your body is straight and relaxed.

Stay in it as long as your consciousness wants, and switch your sides gently by bringing your feet together first.

This asana will develop your back, relieve and stretch the muscles in your legs and open up your lower spine.

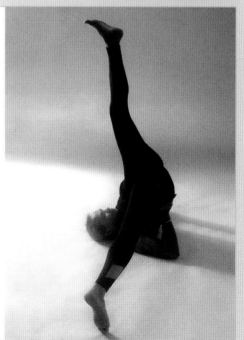

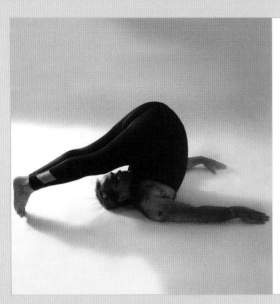

Plough (Hala Asana)

Bring your whole body up into shoulder stand, and if you are totally comfortable, let your legs start to come down over your head.

You can use your palms to support your lower back if you feel a little unstable. When your feet touch the floor you can extend your arms out.

Initially you will feel the stretch in your back and hamstrings. You may also feel a contraction in your stomach and throat. Since the blood will be circulating more in the stomach, chest and neck area, the diseases or imbalances that happen in them will be corrected.

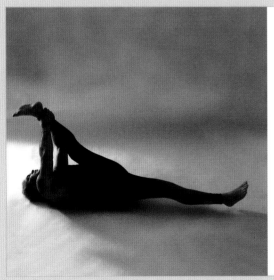

Laying Down Leg Stretch (Supta Padanusthasana)

With your eyes closed, bring either your left or right leg up keeping your knees straight. Hold either the big toe or the calf of the extended leg, relax your body and watch the resistance melt away making room for an incredible stretch. If you relax, it will be hard for you to over-extend yourself.

It is all about hamstrings in this stretch. Hamstrings are the key to balance. This is an excellent stretch for your entire leg.

Body Balancing Qi-gong Movement

Gently bring your palms, facing upwards, below your navel center. Let them rise like some one is lifting them up. There is no effort on your part. Let your arms rise above the heart center, turn around, and come back down again.

This is an excellent exercise to balance both your heart and hara center. Every martial art practice begins and ends with this simple movement. It grounds any excess energy and brings your whole being into a state of oneness. When any Qi-gong movement goes deep within your consciousness you will not be able to tell who is the doer and who is the experiencer. It will merge into one. The slow subtle movements will fill and flow the energy through the body where you will feel strength and center beyond your imagination. The positive impacts are just too many to list.

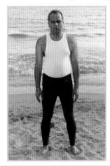 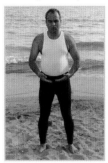 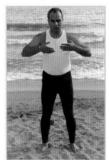 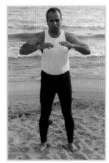 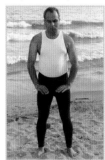 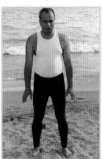

Connecting with the Universal Qi-gong Movement

Have both of your arms face upwards about one and half inches below your navel. Gently let your arms move forward as far as they can go, then move to the side, then come back to the place where they started.

The hara or the third dan-tian is the center of your being. When your whole body relaxes, the energy that is used in your head with thoughts moves and comes to this center. Moving your arms in this pattern, once again lets the energy flow through the body. Each time the energy flows through the body, we feel the oneness and then we forget it and the energy once again becomes stagnant, like air trapped in a house where all the doors and windows are shut. When you open up all the doors and windows, you start to realize that you have been living in a stagnant atmosphere and freshness is your true essence.

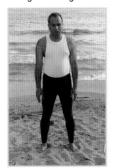 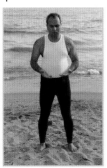 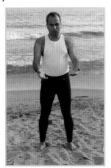 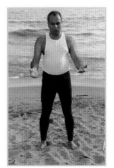 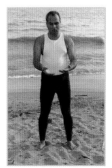 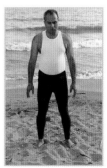

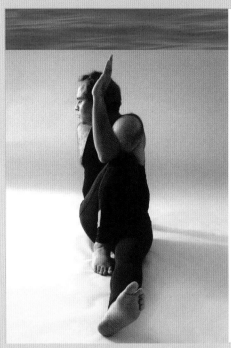

Balance the Water

Sitting Side Abdominal Twist (Marichayasana)

Bring your right foot next to your left thigh. Then bring your right palm behind your spine and place your elbow on the outside of the right knee. The movement should come from your lower spine.

You will feel a tremendous amount of pressure on your stomach and abdominal area. You might find yourself breathing heavily—which is okay. If this happens, then relax your breath. Have no expectations for the stretch.

When you are ready, move to the other side. All asanas that involve lower spinal twist or pressure on the abdominal organs bring about an oneness in the consciousness that is hard to describe.

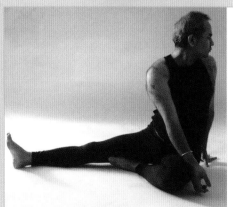

Sitting Lower Spinal Twist

Bring your left foot next to your right thigh. Place your left arm behind your spine and bring your right palm next to your left knee. Twisting from the lower spine, gently go as far as you can possibly go and stay there—totally relaxed. When you are ready, move out and switch sides.

Once again you will see the power of the lower spinal twist that will bring you to a space of oneness. In our daily lives our brain sends signals via the spine to each cell of our body. In the lower spinal twist, the opposite happens; the energy is sent back to the brain or the hypothalamus. This gives an urgently needed break to the brain. The break rejuvenates and vitalizes the brain immensely. With the lower spinal twist, the energy that is in the base of the spine is released and sent to the brain. Bio-chemical endorphins are released in the brain by your pituitary gland. The interesting part is that any slow movement to the lower part of your spine will generate similar response.

Laying down Quad Stretch (Supta Virasana)

Bring your body into a kneeling down position. Gently come to a sitting position like you are sitting on your calf muscles. Next, gently bring both of your hands behind your body and start to slide back. Stop wherever you feel discomfort or pain.

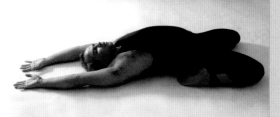

If you can go all the way down to the floor without any pain, then do so. Stay in this position as long as you can. Generally, you will tighten your lower back while doing this exercise. Please let go of this stress to your lower spine and back. You will find that as soon as you release the tension, your whole body will sink to the earth and you will be able to stay in this position forever. This posture will dissipate any fatigue to your legs and body.

This exercise may be a difficult for people who have tight quads and hamstrings. If any part of your leg hurts, while attempting this stretch, please do this stretch one leg at a time. Instead of bringing both of your legs back, bring only one leg back with the other leg extended out.

Extended Leg Stretch (Hasta Padangusthasana)

Sitting down, bring both of your feet together. Raise your left leg up while keeping your knee straight. Hold your foot or your big toe, and touch your chin to your knee.

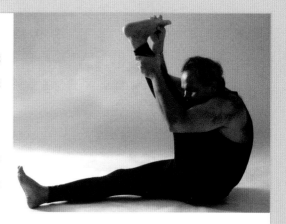

You will feel a stretch through the back of your leg starting from the buttocks to your heel. If your knee is straight, you will feel a deep stretch in your calves.

None of the stretches are going to be easy when you are a beginner. The idea is just to know what your body feels like when you are in these positions.

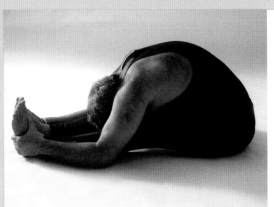

Sitting Forward Bend (Paschimottanasana)

In yoga understanding, the body is divided into four directions: the back is west, front is east, the head is the north and feet are south. The literal translation is west position (because by construction, there is no east left in this stretch). This is one of my favorite exercises.

Close your eyes and bring your feet together while keeping your knees straight. Gently bring your head forward and stop when your body cannot go forward anymore. This asana stretches all of the muscles in the back of your body. If you are new, you will feel a stretch in your lower back. This is because your hamstrings are not fully stretched. Don't push yourself if you have not done stretches before—be gentle. Remember no expectations.

Once you stay in this stretch for a while, you will start to feel it clearly in your hamstrings. This stretch will put a lot of pressure on your stomach and groin area. This is probably the best stretch for balancing the water principle as it works on your pancreas. Stay in it without any expectations and feel the blissfulness.

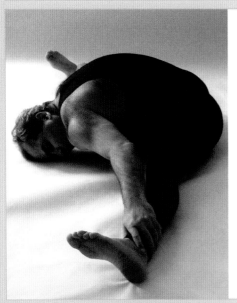

Seated Triangle (Upavistha Konasana)

I call it: "God, I love this stretch!" Bring your legs apart as far as you can while keeping your knees straight. Gently lower your head to the left knee and hold it there as long as you can. Then move to the right knee and hold it as long as you can. Then bring your head forward as far as you can.

You will feel a stretch in your hamstrings, calves, lower back and buttocks. When you have no expectations and come into this silently, you will come to a place in your being that will be sweeter than honey. Your whole body will be stretched out and the oneness will be intoxicating.

Your mind will totally disappear into the vast sky of consciousness.

Managing Expectations and Comparisons

Heaven to Earth Qi-gong movement:

Bring your feet shoulder-width apart with knees slightly bent. Let both of your arms rise up to the side effortlessly like someone is lifting them for you. Let your arms rise all the way up above your head and start to come down through the center of your body all the way below your sex center. Keep repeating this move until you come into a state of total oneness.

You will find that it is very easy to come into a state of oneness with Qi-gong movements. With this movement, you will feel like you are taking an energy shower. With the motion of your hands, you are directing the energy to flow from your head into your feet.

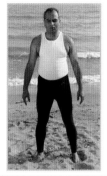 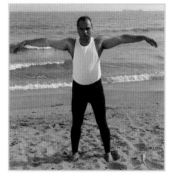 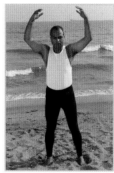 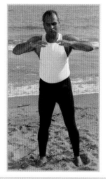 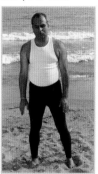

Energy Release Qi-gong Exercise

Bring your feet shoulder width-apart with knees slightly bent. Bring both of your palms to your hips. Gently start to move your body through the lower spine to the left and stay there as long as you can. Then move your body to the right. Do this movement as long as you want.

This movement is incredible in balancing the energy in your body. Sometimes you might feel too much energy which can be overbearing and jittery. This is a simple way to balance that energy out.

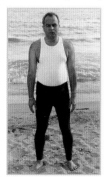 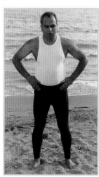 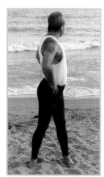 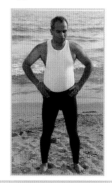 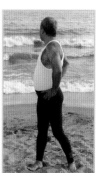 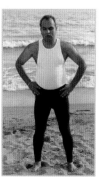

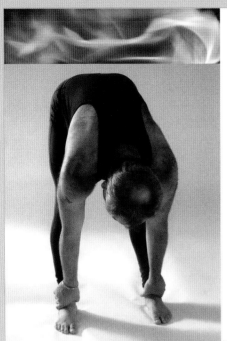

Balance the Fire

Standing Forward Bend (Padangustasana)

Stand straight with your feet about a foot apart and keep your knees straight. Relax your whole body and without any expectation move into a forward bend bringing your head to your knees. Breathe naturally and don't look for anything.

By coming into this asana, you have done your part, now let the divinity do its. You will see that when you relax and have no internal chatter, you are able to go deeper into the stretch like you are reaching further than you could have ever thought. This is yoga where your mind dissolves and you go further and your body is like the measuring stick to detect this phenomenon. Your hamstrings, lower and upper back will get a good stretch improving your balance.

Intense Side Stretch (Parasvottanasana)

Stand straight with your feet 3 to 3.5 feet apart. Move your left foot pointing forward. Bring your right foot in at an angle enough to give your body a good support or base.

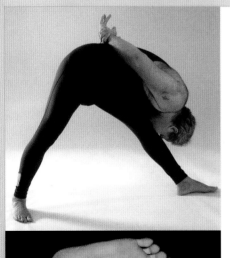

Bring your hands to your back and move your chin forward to your left knee. You will feel an intense stretch in your hamstring, lower and upper back and chest. This is a powerful asana for feeling the two openings or centers on the soles of your feet. If you are totally silent, you will feel them clearly. The exact location is as per the picture shown. This location is also called "the bubbling well" in the Qi-gong methodology. The black dot shows the location of the energy centers.

Triangle Pose (Uttihita Trikonasana)

Stand straight with your feet 3 to 3.5 feet apart. Move your left foot pointing forward. Bring your right foot in at an angle enough to give your body a good support or base.

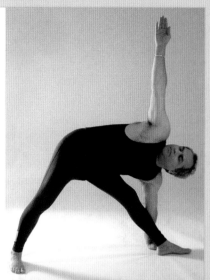

Let both of your arms gently rise up to shoulder length. Without changing your stance, move your upper-body to the left side bringing your palm to either your foot or behind your foot. Keep your knees and arms straight.

If you are totally relaxed you will not want to come out of this posture. Once you disappear in this posture, you will find bliss and silence. When you are ready move your body, do exactly the same things to the other side. Once again disappear into the form and become the formless.

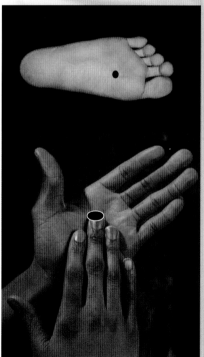

You will intensely stretch your hamstrings and shoulder—not to mention opening up both the energy centers in your palms and soles of your feet as shown in the pictures.

Remember not to look for these locations on the soles of your feet or your palms. When you relax, they will reveal themselves to you. Don't expect to see anything, and it will all come to you.

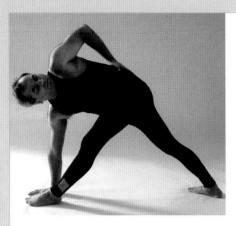

Revolved Triangle (Parivrtta Trikonasana)

Stand straight with your feet 3 to 3.5 feet apart. Move your left foot to point forward. Bring your right foot in at an angle enough to give your body a good support or base.

Let both of your arms gently rise up to your shoulders. Turn your whole body with your right arm coming in front of you and then place it next to the inside of your right foot. You can extend your left arm all the way up or place it like in the picture. Stay in the posture as long as you like and come out when you are ready. Repeat the same directions for the other side. This is a much more intense stretch than the triangle pose as it will stretch parts of your body much more intensely. Your stance is silent and relaxed. Even though you may feel some discomfort, you are not pushing yourself, but being totally relaxed in it. In yoga practice this is how you become non-violent because you learn not to be violent and reactive to your body. On the contrary, you are relaxing in the face of discomfort and not losing consciousness while all of these changes are happening to you. You must have seen, or will be seeing, how having no expectations really takes the edge off in your practice.

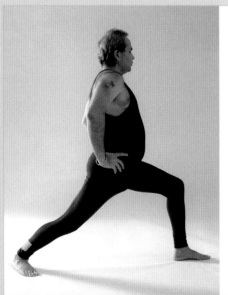

Grounding Asana (Virabhadrasana)

Stand straight with your feet 3 to 3.5 feet apart. Move your left foot to point forward. Bring your right foot in at an angle enough to give your body a good support or base. Bring both of your palms to your hips and move your upper body from the base of the spine to the left. Bend your knee and let it come directly over your left heel.

Stay in this posture as long as you want. When your consciousness is ready, it will bring you out and you can do the same asana to the other side of your body. If you do this posture correctly, you will not be able to feel the weight of your body. The two energy centers on the soles of your feet will become exceptionally clear. However, once again, don't look for them and have no expectation. When the time is right, the energy will reveal itself to you.

Three Heaven Balancing Qi-gong Asana

Stand straight with your feet 3 to 3.5 feet apart. Bring your toes in. Bend both your knees so that you feel like you are sitting on a chair or a stool. Let both of your arms rise up and come over your head, palms upwards. Let your head tilt back like you are able to see the sky. Your lower back should be relaxed releasing any strain in any part of your body.

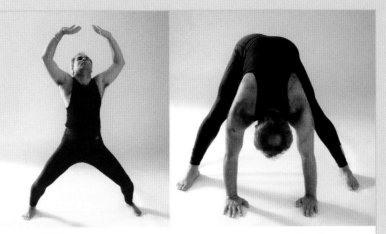

Stay and disappear in this asana. Once you relax, you will have no inclination to come out of this posture. When you are ready, bring your palms to the floor as shown in the picture and stay in it as long as you can. This asana will balance all three centers in the front of your body as shown in the picture. You will feel a balance like you have never experienced before. Once again, this asana will also help you to see the center in the soles of your feet.

Symmetric Angle Asanas (Samakonasana)

Let your feet come as far apart as they can. Place your palms in front of your body for support.

This is an asana where your hamstrings and other leg muscles will get a full intense stretch.

Relax, and let your legs gently move apart. Stop at a point where you cannot go any further. If you are totally relaxed, you will find that you are able to stay in the position for a long time.

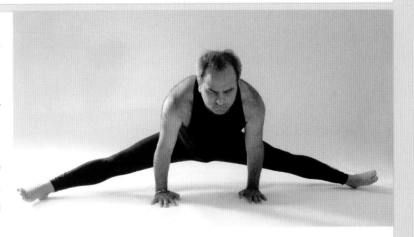

It is interesting that in all the intense stretches, it is necessary to be totally relaxed. It will be impossible to do any of the intense stretches by forcing your body into them.

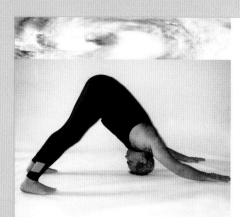

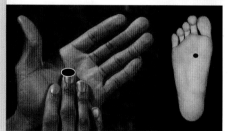

Balance the Air

Downward Facing Dog (Adho Mukh Svanasana)

Bring your body into a push-up position. Keeping your knees straight and your feet flat to the floor, bring the top of your head to the floor.

Stay there as long as you can and watch the energy flow from the soles of your feet out through your palms and top of your head. This asana will show you how the energy flows through the body. You will feel like you are a hollow tube and the energy is passing through you at all times. You will also know clearly that when this energy is blocked, it causes illnesses in the body. A single experience will make all the difference in the world for you to transform forever. Once again you are not expecting to see or looking for any of these things. Be in this position, totally relaxed, without any expectations and watch what will happen. The stretch will be a little tough to do if you are beginner, but your daily practice will show you major improvements. You will feel the stretch all over your body—feet, calves, hamstring, lower back, shoulder, head, and arms. The blood coming into your brain, chest and heart will keep your immune system healthy.

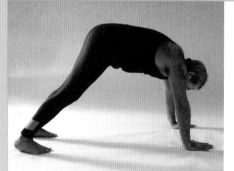

Push-up Position (Svanasana)

Bring your body into a push-up position. Keep your knees straight and your feet flat to the floor. If you keep your feet flat this would be one of the best stretches for your feet and calf muscles.

If you are relaxed and silent, this will significantly strengthen your shoulders and build upper-body strength. The strength of your body is not built by building bulky muscles. It is felt when the energy flows through your body. When your body is totally grounded, you will feel like nobody can shake you. The subtle moves of Qi-gong will show you that it is the energy that flows through you and that is sustaining everything in and around you. Did you ever wonder what keeps all the stars and planets in their orbits and their place? Why don't they just run into each other or fall down in a pile? The planets and stars are all in a state of yoga doing their own orbital Qi-gong movements.

Staff Pose (Chaturanga Dandasana)

Come into a push-up position and gently lower your body to two inches away from the floor. Another way to do this asana will be by lying flat on the floor and lifting your body up about two inches from the floor.

This asana will strengthen your wrists, arms, chest and shoulders. It will put intense pressure on them. Your breathing might get faster, which is fine, just relax your body and it will start to come back into a rhythm. Once again, it is a different situation for your body, and it is going to reveal all types of things associated with it.

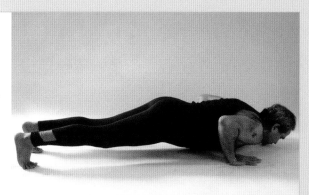

Cobra (Bhujangasana)

Lie flat to the floor with your palms next to your face and shoulders. Gently press your palms to the floor and let your upper-body rise up and away from the floor. You will feel an intense stretch on your lower back.

This is a powerful exercise for your lower back. Do the best you can without exerting too much pressure. If you have no expectations, you will be able to see all the benefits of this pose.

Once you totally relax your body, you will have a hard time coming out of this asana.

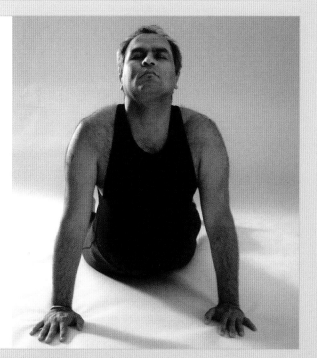

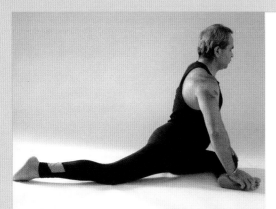

Pigeon Pose (Kapotasana)

Bring yourself into a push-up position, then gently bring your left foot forward and place it perpendicular to your body. Follow the picture for the exact location of your leg. Keep your upper body straight. Eventually you will be able to bring your body back.

Once your body feels totally relaxed, and your consciousness wants to move on, then switch sides and repeat the asana. If you are new, your leg may not be perpendicular and you will feel an intense stretch on your back and buttocks. When you find yourself being challenged, don't struggle with it, it will only make things more difficult. Over a period of time, you will feel at home in this asana (situation) as well. You will feel an intense stretch in your buttocks and back. If you come from a space of no-expectation, you will not have to fight with your body. This is because with no expectations, your mind will have disappeared—this is the state of yoga where only your consciousness and body remain.

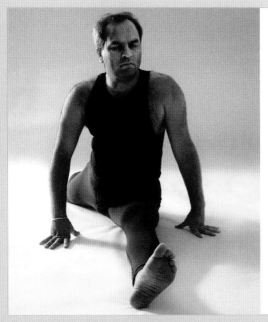

Splits (Hanumanasana)

Come into the pigeon pose as shown previously and let the leg in front of your body slide forward. You are making a right angle with your upper body and your legs.

When you are done with one side, repeat the asana with the other side to keep your body in balance. Needless to say, this is a very intense stretch. It will take some time for you to become totally comfortable in it. It is in an intense stretch that it will become clear to you if you have understood the fundamentals of Yoga. If you are not relaxed and have expectations, this will be an impossible asana. Asana means a sculpture. It means that your body is so relaxed in the posture that it has become a sculpture. A person looking at you from the outside cannot tell if you are alive because the stillness in your asana is so deep and profound.

Managing Expectations and Comparisons

Camel Posture (Ustrasana)

Kneel down using pads underneath your knees to avoid any discomfort and damage. Bring your palms to either your lower back or to the soles of your feet as shown.

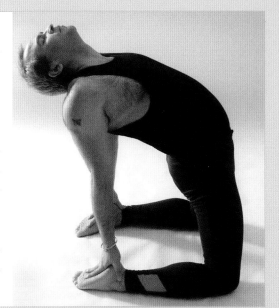

This asana will stretch and open your chest, face, quad muscles and all the muscles in the front of your body. You will also feel a stretch in your shoulders and arms. The real beauty of this stretch is that it opens up the lower part of the spine so that the energy can move into the center of your brain. While in this asana check your lower back and buttocks; you may find them to be frozen. When we encounter a challenging situation, our first and natural response is to freeze. This is the block to your transformation. The moment you realize that this block is the creation of your fear, it will automatically let go and you will be able to relax into the asana. This posture shows you the power of a yoga stretch. In one posture, your entire body is stretched and relaxed.

Camel Posture II (Ustrasana II)

This is a variation of the previous asana. The only difference being that one hand comes to the floor while the other rises up into the sky.

The stretch to your lower back is going to be more intense than the previous asana. Also, this asana will also open up and strengthen your shoulders. Repeat the streatch on the other side.

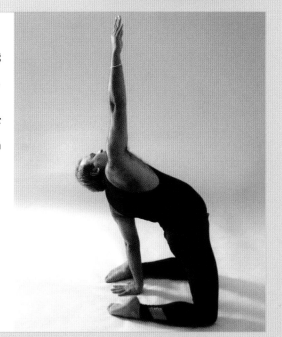

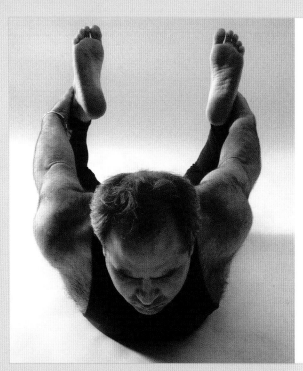

Bow Posture (Dhanurasana)

Facing down, bring your body flat to the floor. Bend your knees, hold your ankles and kick your legs back. This will lift your head up and you will feel a stretch all over your body especially in the front. Your breathing might increase since there is a lot of pressure being put on your lungs, heart and kidneys.

This is a great abdominal stretch because it is only in this stretch that you put direct pressure on your stomach and all the internal abdominal organs. This stretch will also increase your overall body flexibility. Once again there is a possibility that you might tighten your lower back and leg muscles. Be aware of it and as soon as see that it is happening, relax, release the tension and let the divine energy flow through your body.

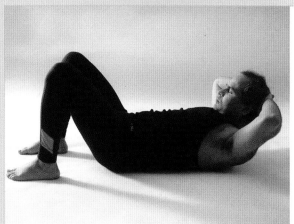

Sit-up (Navasana I)

Lie down flat on your back and bring your palms behind your head. Bend your knees and place your feet on the floor. Gently raise your head up and hold it for as long as you can. Bring your head down and lay there for few seconds and then once again repeat the process. Lift and hold at least five times.

This is a simple, yet powerful, exercise to bring the energy into your third Dan Tian (the main energy hub in your body). Your core strength and consciousness is directed by this center. Come into it with no expectations and you will find that you are both gentle and firm while in this position. All sit-ups are excellent for your back and stomach.

East Plank Stretch (Purvottanasana)

If you recall, the front of the body is identified as the east side of the body. Hence, this position is called the east plank stretch.

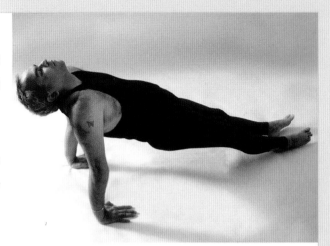

Sitting on the floor with your legs and knees straight, place your arms to the side and push on the palms to lift your body up while keeping your knees and legs straight.

You will feel pressure on your wrist, arms, shoulders, stomach and feet. Stay in this asana for as long as you can.

Upward Bow I (Urdhava Dhanurasana I)

Lie down flat on the floor and bend both your knees and your elbows while your palms face inwards.

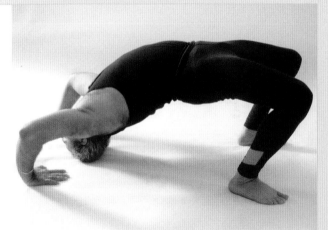

When ready, apply pressure with both your feet and palms and lift your body up and place your head on the floor. Don't put pressure on your head. Your weight should be borne by your stomach, lower back, legs and arms.

This is a strenuous posture to be attempted only after you feel you have a lot of strength and flexibility in your body. This posture stretches the whole front part of your body and builds strength in your arms, legs and lower back.

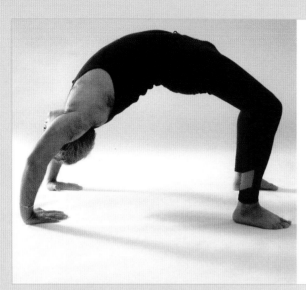

Upward Bow II (Urdhava Dhanurasana II)

This asana is the extension of the previous one where your body needs enough strength and flexibility to lift completely up. This asana will give a complete, thorough stretch to your entire body.

Once again, be aware of your lower back and stomach as you tighten it. By tightening these muscles, you will strain them and other muscles in the body. Once you relax them, you will feel an incredible stretch in your body. This is an excellent stretch if you want to increase both blood and energy circulation in your body. This is the best stretch for balancing Vyana vayu (main air circulatory principle).

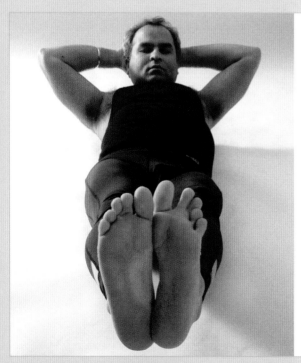

Half Boat Posture (Ardha-Navasana)

This asana is a more intense version of the sit-up. Lying on your back, flat on the floor, bring your palms behind your head. Then lift both your legs and head up together. Hold it for as long as you can. You will feel a lot of pressure on your stomach because you will be using your stomach and back muscles to lift your legs up.

This asana will build both your stomach and back muscles. Do as many repetitions as possible. I don't like to tell you how much and how long to hold your asana. How long you hold an asana depends upon how strong and relaxed you are. If I tell you how long to hold it, or how many repetitions to do, I will be building an expectation in you.

Managing Expectations and Comparisons

Lotus Position (Padmasana)

There are two ways to do this asana:

Easy Way

To bend your right knee and bring your foot next to your groin, then bend your left knee and place the left foot on top of the right.

Challenging Way

To bend and place the right foot on the left thigh and then place the left foot on the right thigh.

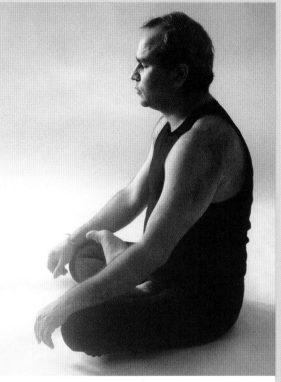

You can start with the easy way first and then as your flexibility improves do the second, more-challenging asana. Only when you are able to sit in the more-challenging asana, will you realize what it means to be sitting straight. Your spine and shoulders will be straight, your lumbar will be curved, and your body will not spend any energy to keep your upper body in a balance.

It is in this posture only that the base of your spine will be in correct alignment with the earth for the earth energy to rise up through the spine and come into the center of the brain. That is the reason why it is called lotus position or (padmasana) because it is in this posture that the thousand-petal lotus in the center of your brain will open up.

Balancing the Earth and Heaven Energy-Qi-gong Movement

Have both of your palms face upwards at your third dan-tian (one inch below the navel). Gently let the left palm rise up facing upwards towards the sky while the right palm, facing downwards, moves towards the earth. When your palms reach their maximum distance then let them flip and move in the opposite direction. It is a very simple move which will feel like you are swimming in consciousness. This is very close to freestyle swimming; the only difference is that the movements are happening to you without any expectations.

When the palm rises from below, it will feel like the energy is moving from the earth into the body and out through the top of the head. When the palm moves from above the head it will feel like the energy is moving from the sky into your body and out into the earth. A relaxed two to three minutes with this move will show you more than you can read in a thousand books.

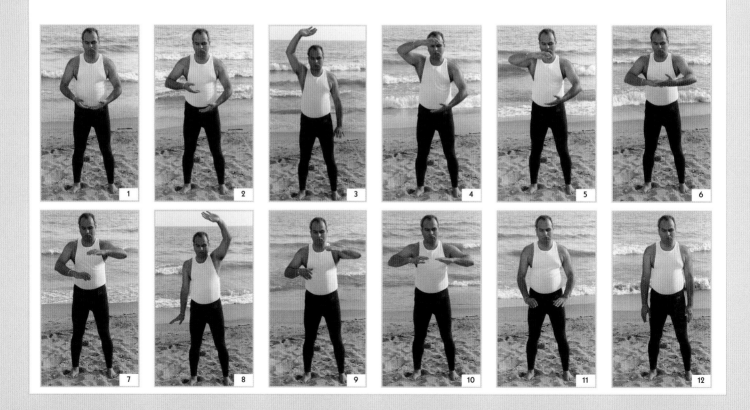

When In the Real World:

Your health is like a bank account; when you put money into your account, the amount in your account increases, and vice versa. Your body is the bank where you deposit the energy (money) into it. All the stress, sickness and activities are like the withdrawals that you make against the account. If you have less money (energy) in your account (body), you will be overdrawn. All the things that happen to you when you are overdrawn in your checking account will apply in your body as well.

Deposits:

Exercising everyday will be the biggest deposit that you can make into your account. Exercise reduces both physiological and psychological stress. It fills and circulates the whole body with energy.

The type of food that you eat is also a deposit. If you eat food that will take more time and energy to digest, then your net deposit is going to be less. Imagine going to your local bank and depositing a check that is written from a foreign account. Your bank is going to put a hold on the money, and charge you a fee to do the process. This is what happens when you eat foods that are not easily digestible by your system. Your body has to do many things to convert it into energy and in the process, it loses energy.

Withdrawals:

Stress is the biggest withdrawal that you will make. It keeps your body constantly overdrawn because during stress, you don't deposit much and your withdrawals are huge. To meet your withdrawal needs, you have to take a loan from your kidney or your heart or your intestines.

Once you take a loan from them, you have to repay back or else they will go bankrupt—which could mean kidney failure, hypertension, heart attack or ulcerated colitis.

All of the sicknesses, which include any outbreaks of bacteria or viruses that might happen to you, would be a withdrawal from your immune system. Your body takes away from your immune system (health reserve) to fight the disease. This is like an accident that might happen to you while driving your car and someone hits you. If you have strong immune system, with lots of reserve, you will be able to pay for big accidents, however if you have poor immune system, then you will be bankrupt.

If you spend too much energy in all of these activities such as job, community service or exercise, without knowing and keeping a balance, then once again, you will be overdrawn.

Your health is the balance between your deposits and withdrawals. Your immune system (ojas) is the reserve (cushion) that you will need at all times to fend off any accident that might happen. A rule of thumb to lower your withdrawals is to cut your expenses due to stress to zero, and spend half of what you bring in and shortly you will become a healthy millionaire. Your outside wealth is great, but if you don't have your sanity and your physical health to enjoy it, then it will become a source of frustration. In becoming this millionaire you have become a millionaire forever because no matter where you go, or where you are, you will be living in a state of abundance.

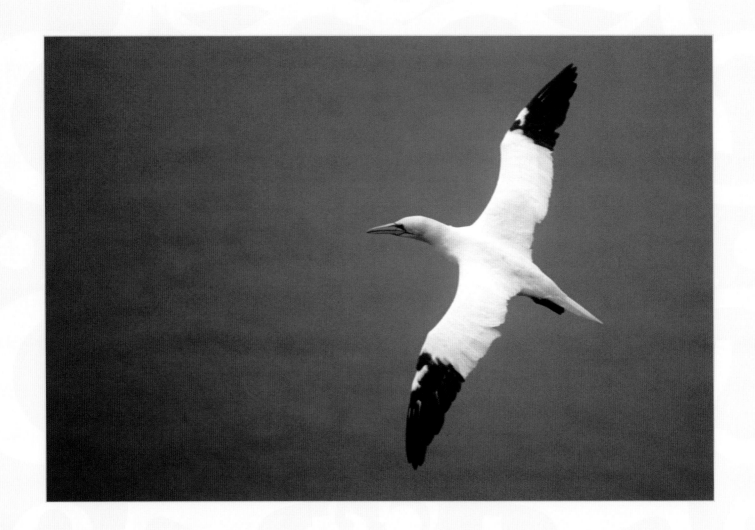

Giving myself to the sky
I let my spirit fly
Like a bird on the wing
I'm letting go
High with the clouds above
I disappear in love
With a song in my heart
I dance with the wind
Into the light
Like a moth to a flame
Closer and closer
Burning so bright (Ever so bright).

Anand Milarepa (Mystical poet)

I arrived in America on January 6th, 1986 in a total daze. I did not know many people or the culture or what to expect. Reflecting back, it seems like jumping off a cliff with my eyes closed, leaving everything. I had never even seen snow up until then. I attended Akron University in Ohio where I eventually completed two M.A. degrees, one in International Economics and the other in Statistics.

Initially, going to a university was a lot of hard work, but towards the end it seemed to get easier. The real challenge was living alone. I had never lived away from my family and had not really known anybody in America. I did not know that I had arrived in the country of the lonely. There were two ways that I knew how not to be alone—alcohol and relationships. You must be thinking, "What bad choices,"—especially if you have been there and done that. I couldn't wait to go to the bars on Thursday, Friday and Saturday every week—which, of course, led to drinking problems. And the relationships that I had did not materialize into anything meaningful.

One day, sometime in the summer of 1988, I realized that I liked to be drunk all the time. It did not matter if it was afternoon, evening or night. In Alcoholics Anonymous (AA) terminology this is called a "moment of clarity." I had this moment on my own, even though I was not aware of AA. Looking back upon it, it was that day that I started to move away from alcohol. However, giving up alcohol does not solve any problems, it only exposes them. Only now, I couldn't go back and intoxicate myself. Now that I had gone through this journey of being drunk and being sober, I could watch other people get drunk. It wasn't fun anymore, so the bar scene started to be less attractive.

The thorn of loneliness was still there in my consciousness and was making the pain worse. I would get involved with the first person I met. Most of these people had not had good, stable lives themselves. I found out later, that with few exceptions, this was the "American Way." The family system has disintegrated under the stress of making ends meet, rugged individualism and unawareness. In all this fog, chaos and commotion I was searching for something to ease the pain of constant loneliness and thoughts. Always being engaged in expectations, virtual reality and Type B thoughts without any end in sight does not help. It is like living in some place where you almost never see the sun shine. So the day you do see the big red ball in the sky, you want to run into the house because you don't know what to do with it.

All my life in India, I had heard people saying that meditation was a good thing. So in 1989 I joined mantra meditation group where a "Guru" gave me five words to repeat while focusing on my third eye. These five words were given in secret—not to be shared with anybody else. So you cannot start your own following, I guess? I woke up every morning at 3 AM and repeated the words without any guidance. After having done it for 3 months or so, I realized that my whole body would become stiff especially my knees, my back and my legs, which would go to sleep. I was only 25 years old and in fairly athletic condition at that time, so I was physically capable of doing the meditation. I asked several people involved with the group about the problem and they did not know what to do either. Some of them acknowledged that they had had the same problem too. It was like a tree that they were holding on to in the midst of the storm that was happening in their head. The worst thing was that I was not able to make any progress with this type of meditation technique due to the lack of guidance and understanding.

In the mean time, the common understanding was that anger and lust were two worst things that can happen to you and should be avoided at any cost. This was a toughie. I found myself angry all the time and definitely more sexual since I was trying to repress it. Not a good thing. It made any kind of stillness impossible. So I gradually started to look for other things, but felt guilty that I was abandoning my adopted "Guru."

One day, at a party, I was having a philosophical discussion with my friend W. He asked if I had heard anything by Rajneesh (now known as Osho). I said "No, and I am NOT INTERESTED! I am looking to calm my mind and come to a state of meditation, so what do I need a sex guru for?" He insisted that I should listen to a discourse tape by Osho in Hindi commenting on the Maha-geeta by Astavakra (an enlightened mystic) on meditation. So very reluctantly, not to be impolite, I accepted the tape that sat in my car for two weeks collecting dust. Being in a stormy relationship with no peace in sight, I finally decided to listen to the tape. In first 15 minutes, I don't know what happened. He said that one has to understand to transcend and not to repress anything. Everything he said made more sense to me than anything I had ever heard up until that point. So I started to get more into what he had to say about everything. I bought books and tapes by him and listened to them all the time. I started to meditate as per his instruction. I experimented with both Dynamic and Kundalini meditation, two of his most famous techniques. I started to feel more relaxed and have a better idea about things in more esthetic and natural way. I started to practice yoga asanas with a local teacher as well.

The yoga asana classes were based on a liberal Iyengar style, rooted and focused on the body alone. I was interested in feeling any kind of relief from the storm in my head. I felt wonderful in my body after the class, but it would not stay very long. Soon, I was back to myself again (alone with a storm). So I decided to move away from exercises, focus entirely on meditation and read as much as I could. I started to experiment with many types of meditative techniques as per Osho's suggestion. I practiced for six years and started to have a taste of the space called "meditation" or "yoga."

In 1997, I stopped reading anything—including Osho's books. I found that I knew what I needed to do, and had a good idea what it felt like. Reading had served its purpose, but where I wanted to go, only energy could go there. It was time to give up that last crutch (of reading). I was devoting more time to meditative practices.

Since starting the journey in 1990, every morning after I woke up from sleep, I would sit in silence for any length of time. Looking back, I find that this was probably the most effective thing that I did. The key was consistency. Every day means every day. Over a period of time, I became conscious of the activity in my mind and the everyday situations that happened there—Type B's, but I did not know, back then, what to do with them.

Any typical morning, I would sit down comfortably in silence, thoughts would appear, and I would find a conversation happening. I was very much a part of it. Then they would leave, and there would be silence. Then another thought would come and the same pattern would be repeated all over again: "virtual reality." About an hour or so into this, I would feel a little tired, lie down and enter a deep state of meditative sleep. By the time I woke up, I would have to get ready and go to work. Osho always talked about sitting silently and doing nothing. Back then, it was easier said than done.

The meditation techniques gave me a temporary relief from the storm, but I could never find a way to not have any thoughts or Type B situations. It is like driving a car with both of your eyes closed and missing an accident when you intermittently happen to open one eye. The intermittent opening of one eye is the time you spend in meditation or are aware. Well, I could not be sitting in meditation all the time. Obviously I had to work and live my life. This is the struggle that every seeker goes through. Perhaps that is why Siddhartha had to leave his kingdom to become Buddha. Like Siddartha, what do you want, your sanity or a kingdom? The answer lies in what are you closest to. If you are close to your kingdom, you will never leave. If you are close to your insanity and want relief, you will leave to find your peace. There was progress, as I could feel the peace, but it seemed temporary.

The daily practice of meditation kept me going with new experiences in my consciousness and mind on daily basis. In 1997 I started to teach meditation techniques once a week. I facilitated only meditation techniques prescribed by Osho because they were the only ones that I knew to be effective, and I had worked with them for eight years. The techniques were very powerful, but very physical, so many people were unable to do them. In addition, many people did not understand how they needed to be done. The "let-go" and totality are the keys to any meditative technique. If I had had the understanding and experience of "let-go," then I would not need the technique anyway, would I? It is a Catch 22 situation. I found out that all meditative techniques are like someone telling you that place you are looking for is between two cities, but you don't have a concrete address. Now you have to find this place while you are half asleep, with traffic moving from all directions, and no one can give you clear instructions. So everybody was on their own and there was no way to tell if the meditation techniques were really working. It seemed almost impossible for me to get a new student to any level of understanding.

The best way, I realized, was not to instruct in meditative techniques, but to bring the students to the experience of "here and now." Instead of giving them the address, I would take the time to bring them to the address or the experience. If I did not have it, then I would not be able to explain it either. If this was going to happen, it had to happen on its own and existence would have to support it. So I started teaching yoga and Qi-gong again. Yoga became a language of conveying silence. I could communicate like a silent dance with whoever was there with me at the time. I started to see that after each class, we came to an experience of oneness. In addition, my body was well integrated into my spiritual practice. Before this time, they were artificially separated. I had to go to the gym to work out and then I did my meditation. The Qi-gong made the entire practice of relaxation very easy, and I could feel the energy all the time. The mind and the chatter would fall away. I would feel like I was standing in water and had become the water. This I found to be the healing energy. Not only was I able to communicate and bring my friends to the essence, but also our bodies were relaxed, exercised and healed all at the same time. In fact, in the ancient texts, the definition of yoga is given as "A process of re-integration".

The yoga practice was going fine for a while, until I discovered that my body would get stiff whenever thoughts were there. So if I am standing in "downward-facing dog" pose, but my consciousness is busy with a Type B thought, all my energy is in the Type B thought. I would essentially be doing two things: the pose and trying to solve this real life problem. Obviously, that is not the right pose to solve the problem at hand. My body felt good and relaxed after a yoga session, but the Type B thoughts came back as soon as I was back in the world.

More understanding of the state of yoga was needed. Yoga asanas helped with quieting the Type A thoughts and rejuvenating the body so that the Type B's could become clearer. My consciousness also started to become clearer and many of the more intricate workings of my mind were revealed. For example, if you could get silent all of a sudden for two days that would be great, but you need to know why you became silent. However, if you find a way to be silent all the time, and use the mind only to communicate and do Type A kinds of things, then you have something. This happened to me one morning in my daily sitting—something just lifted off of me, and for the first time, I discovered the transient nature of thoughts and how they were nothing but reflections on the consciousness. In other words, they never touch your consciousness.

I immediately started to put this into practice, and identified that there were essentially two types of thoughts: the ones that don't engage you and are convenience thoughts, and the ones that engage you (Type B thoughts). I kept working on myself for some time, to make sure that this was not a trick that my mind was playing. Then I discovered that as soon as I became aware of an engaging thought in my consciousness, the thought became completely inactive and started to die. I saw this over and over again and realized that each time a new thought came into my consciousness, it was less and less powerful. Within a week, I had no Type B thoughts. I knew very well what would happen when a Type B thought came into my consciousness—it would be a total waste of energy with lingering after-effects.

With only Type A thoughts there, the silence and feeling of oneness in the yoga classes that I taught got even deeper. I was curious about how this would work with my friends and students, whom I found were also afflicted with Type B thoughts. So I instructed all of my students and friends on how to spot a Type B thought and see it disappear. To my delight, I have received very good responses from everyone, which led me to further experiment with it.

Once the Type B thoughts subsided, the energy that was released from them went into other parts of my body and mind. The next big breakthrough was when one day while I was in my yoga practice I discovered that I was totally separated from the thoughts; they were moving, but I was not affected by them. This made it absolutely clear that there is something within me that was far away from thoughts, and that I didn't have to pay any attention to them. Having realized this phenomenon, I wanted to create a practice for others who may not have had this experience. After all, this is what we all are trying to do—not to be impulsive to thoughts. The best and easiest thing to do was to create a dark room to simulate the mind and use a flashlight to simulate the thoughts. Then by moving a flashlight around, while not focusing on the light you will learn to not focus on the light. This I hoped would undo what was happening inside our minds. I tried this with several of my students and it worked and they had an even deeper experience of consciousness.

The oil lamp technique from Chapter 3 helps in moving the energy from the soles of your feet to your head—you will actually feel the energy moving. Once the energy moves, it relaxes the whole body.

This technique brought about a lot of changes; the most significant was that I was not focusing on thoughts during the day. This further enhanced awareness and alertness. In this alertness, I started to sense how comparative people were around me. I found out that I was constantly comparing, and this was a source of disturbance to my consciousness. Whether I needed to or not, I always automatically did it anyway. This I found caused hell in my life. Then I discovered that I was always trying to compare to something that I was expecting to see. This led to the discovery on how expectations impacted my life. We all know about expectations, and we use the word about 50 times in a day, but we don't understand the impact they have on our life.

When I realized their impact, I was just stunned and then I started to see changes in my asana and movement practice. I was just amazed at the experience of oneness—like I was doing yoga for the first time—like I had never ever tasted the space of yoga before. From then on, every class that I taught, the first thing I told my students was to not expect anything from this class. All you can do is create an environment, but you cannot expect anything or you will miss it by disturbing the process. Doing yoga and Qi-gong exercises is the best way to learn the power of non-expectation and non-comparison because you will feel the impact instantaneously. If you have expectations, it will be very hard for you to relax and when you come with no expectations, you will get showered with divinity.

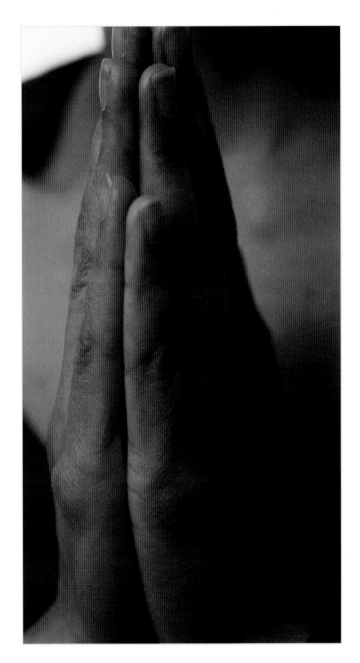

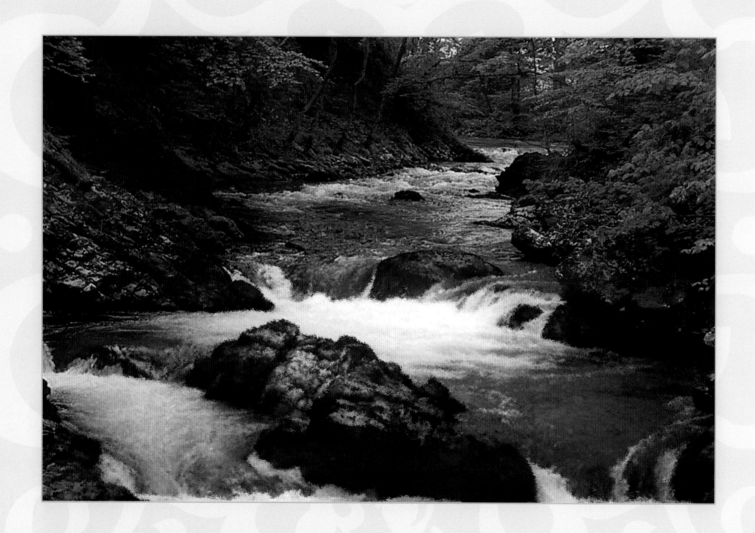

I ask for a moment's indulgence to sit by thy side.
The works that I have in hand I will finish afterwards.

Away from the sight of thy face my heart knows no rest nor respite,
and my work becomes an endless toil in a shoreless sea of toil.

Today the summer has come at my window with its sighs and murmurs;
and the bees are playing their minstrels at the court of the flowering grove.

Now it is time to sit quiet,
face to face with thee,
and to sing dedication of life in this silent and overflowing leisure.

Gitanjali (Gurudev Rabindranath Tagore)

When you drive a car, the most important thing is the road in front of you. If you cannot see the road, no matter how good a driver you are, you will not be very effective. When you are driving, there are times when the road twists and turns, and other times when it can be straight for miles. You move your car based on the road you see, and your every move is directed by this reference. When you have no reference, you have no way of knowing when to turn or when to keep straight. There is nothing but chaos. In yoga, your reference is consciousness. When you lose this reference, then it is anybody's guess what you are following. When you are not connected to the road for whatever reason, you can imagine the danger. The same is true in any other situation.

To follow things blindly is similar to being disconnected to the road. Stress and chatter can be so overwhelming that we will go to any lengths just to get a break. Desperately trying any means to achieve the unclear end causes more problems and a lot of confusion. Some of the means that we use are food, sex, drugs, alcohol, money, prestige, or power. The unknown destination is actually freedom from the chatter of the mind, which is always happening to us. Needless to say, none of the methods that have been listed are going to work because what we are trying to solve is unsolvable. We fail to realize that putting food, sex, or drugs into our system will only disturb our system further, rather than bringing it to a state of stillness. However, in doing these things, we get occupied, lose consciousness of the chatter and get a break from it. This break is what you were looking for, and you do achieve it by doing these things, so you think that they might be the doors.

This has become the state of the world today, especially in the West, where things are moving at a speed that is faster than one can comprehend. We don't realize that the faster we move, the chatter will increase proportionately, but we have no time to figure that part out. The goal is to move away from the present moment, because in the present moment, there is nothing but chatter and stress. That is why we keep ourselves occupied and our schedules full. It is even hard to go on a vacation because we don't know how to relax when we arrive at the beach or the mountain.

This unconsciousness of the present is what robs us of our life. Then, whether we are dead or alive does not make much of a difference because the essence or quality of life is missing. If your consciousness is missing, it is like saying that the sun is missing in our solar system. There will be no solar system. All the spiritual practices in the world try to indicate or bring us to the present. Some are more effective then others, depending on how much emphasis they put on consciousness. A religion will be effective if all of its effort is put into making its practitioners conscious and eliminating any of their virtual realities. If a religion makes you unconscious or adds to your virtual reality, then it will not be very helpful to you. On the contrary, it will be extremely harmful.

How can yoga help?

Yoga is one such conscious/aware spiritual practice in the world. There are two very significant things that it clearly brings out:

1) Combining the body and the consciousness. In yoga, your body is your temple and consciousness is the godliness that flows through it. The exercise part is like cleaning the temple, decorating the temple, and praying in the temple. The consciousness part is the divinity. The interesting thing is that both the body and consciousness are alive. The body becomes totally alive when it merges and mingles with the consciousness. In this merging, a beautiful dance starts to happen between them. This dance is the definition of love or balance. Another way to look at it would be like seeing the relationship between a house and the air that is in and all around the house. Think of a house as the body and the air as the consciousness or air that one breathes. If, for some reason, no air can either enter or leave a particular house, then no one will be able to live in it. Death will occur.

2) Yoga gives you a framework of reference. Say you are walking in a park and you lose balance and fall. You realize that you lost balance, dust off, maybe find the cause of your fall and get back to your walking again. The key here is the realization that you lost balance, because if you

did not have that, you would still be on the ground. Your internal realization of balance is your framework of reference; when you move away from it, it brings you right back. Consciousness is the framework of your reference and the practice of yoga brings out this reference. So when you start to move away from it, it will automatically bring you back into the state. You will not have to go completely wrong and find out when it is too late. There is no question of living in sin or in virtue; you are living in a state of the present.

Seeds of Wisdom

Yoga, as we know today, is a part of an ancient methodology to understand and live life according to the laws of nature. Many great seers, mystics and enlightened beings have added to this system over the years. However, one such enlightened being, the sage Patanjali, has been credited to have synthesized all the yogic teachings so that a practitioner can get all the information they need to reach to their consciousness.

The title of the book "Yoga Sutras" means yoga seeds or essence which cannot be any clearer. They certainly are seeds because they will be meaningful only if planted in your consciousness. The seeds are magical because they also help you clear your consciousness and set it free. The essence of each chapter can be clearly understood with an illustration of burning incense. There are four things that happen when you burn incense and they all happen simultaneously:

- The making of the incense.
- The actual process of burning the incense with fire.
- The ash that is left behind once the incense burns.
- The fragrant smell in the form of smoke that rises up to the sky.

Fragrance of Consciousness

- In "Yoga Sutras," the first chapter, Samadhi pada, gives a description of consciousness. It gives information on what it feels like to be in the final stage. In our incense example, it would be like describing the incense stick itself.

•The chapter on Sadhana pada gives all the information on the steps that need to be taken for transformation.   Literal translation of the word Sadhana would be diligent practice with focus. It would be like giving information on how to light the incense.

•The third chapter, Vibhuti pada, describes what is left behind or (acquired and released) once the transformation occurs. In the case of the incense, it is the ashes that are accumulated or left behind from burning the incense—the by-product of the process.

•In the final chapter or Kaivalya pada, (which literally means one and only) he describes the essence of consciousness. It is like describing the fragrance and stillness of the smoke rising from the incense once you have totally experienced it.

The Journey

The Yoga Sutras of Patanjali are the guidelines and map of the process of yoga. They tell you clearly what is required for your journey and what will you see as you approach your destination. If you are planning to take a trip, you want to find out all the details beforehand, such as: the weather at your destination, places to stay, traveling and lodging costs and many more things. In addition, if you are traveling by car or a train, you want to know what you can expect to see so that you know you are going in the right direction.

Eight steps are outlined by Patanjali: Yama, Niyama, Asana, Pranayama, Prathyhara, Dharna, Dhyana, and Samadhi. These steps can be divided into two groups of four steps. The first four steps can be thought of as things required for the journey. The last four can be thought of as things that will happen to you when you are actually taking the journey.

The Eight-Step Process as per Sage Patanjali:

• Yama are qualities required of an individual to embark on the journey: non-violence (ahimsa), truth (satya), non-stealing (asteya), being in love with divinity (bramcharya or brama-ki-charya) and non-coveting (aparigraha).

• Niyama are the overall requirements: purity (saucha), contentment (santosha), ardour or penance (tapas), study of the self (svadhyaya) and dedication to consciousness (isvara pranidhana).

• Asana are the techniques that will keep your body in balance. These are the stretching and strength-building exercises that will help to clear your body of toxins and other diseases. Your posture, endurance and immune system will be improved and your body will become revitalized.

• Pranayama are the breathing techniques that show you the subtle relationship between the body and the universal consciousness. Pranayama build and release the energy required in your body. When we bring this process into a balance, then we are able to live fully.

• Prathyhara is a state of no-mind. This state happens to you when you have no expectations or no comparisons. It is the first step towards knowing your essence. It is like when the sun just starts to rise on the horizon and you see a brilliant orange or saffron-color light. This is a state where you will have long periods of time without any chatter or disturbance. The first five chapters are techniques to bring you to this state.

• Dharna is the state of becoming. It is a state that can happen to you when you listen to the music by your favorite artist or composer. It is the state that can happen to you when you are holding a new-born child in your arms or looking at a beautiful piece of art. You get filled up with some unknown combining force that takes away all your distractions. The literal meaning of the word dharna means to become. It is also a state of "Bhairava" which means where all the fragmented energies come together and move with a strong force. You can think of this state as a huge fire that burns with strong blaze.

• Dhyana is an absolute state of alertness or focus. In short it is an undisturbed state of alertness.

• Samadhi is an egoless or non-dual state where the process of duality has ended.

Functionally, the eight steps can be also thought as a purification process. For example, you have a large container of dirty water and you want to purify the water so that it is drinkable. The water can be thought of as your consciousness and the dirt is all the psychological (mental) and physical blocks or challenges that you might have. The first two steps (Yama and Niyama) in the purification process are removing big stones or pieces of debris in the water. The second two steps (Asana and Pranayama) can be thought of as removing any harmful chemicals or heavy metals. The third two steps (Prathyhara and Dharna) can be thought of as removing harmful bacteria, germs or other organisms. Once all these are removed, your water becomes drinkable (Dhyana and Samadhi). Otherwise you might get fatally sick from drinking the glass of water.

The first two steps (Yama and Niyama) are required to clear the consciousness of any psychology. The next two steps (Asana and Pranayama) are required to balance and rejuvenate the body. The next two steps (Prathyhara and Dharna) are where more subtle disturbances to the consciousness are removed and where it becomes absolutely still. The last two steps are the transformation of the consciousness into its essence. It makes sense that the psychological aspects have to be covered first in a human being because they are the biggest source of disturbance, followed by disturbance through the imbalances in the body and by even more subtle disturbances in the consciousness.

The purification process needs to be understood very clearly for you to be able to know how it works. You will need to know what constitutes a clear or purified glass of water. Only then can you measure the contamination in your glass of drinking water, identify it and its sources and take steps to correct them. You will also be able to avoid any type of contamination that might even possibly happen. Even more importantly, if you see dirty water anywhere, you will be able to identify its source and suggest what needs to be done right away.

To translate it into your yoga practice, this would mean that you would need to know your clear or clean state up front, which would be the state of

Dhyana and Samadhi. Once you know this state of clarity, you will very easily know the sources of contamination.

Going back to the "taking the trip" example, if you know where you want to go, you will be able to prepare yourself properly. If you are going to a beach, you will pack your bags with things that you will need at the beach. Similarly, if you know the space of Dhyana and Samadhi, you will only do things that will take you or keep you in that state. For example, nobody will have to tell you to be a non-violent person, because you know very well that with violence, you will disturb the state of Dhyana and Samadhi.

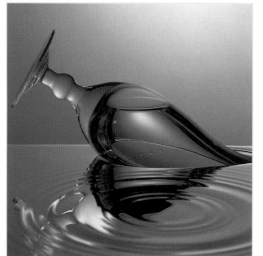
The container and the content become one

You cannot be a person who lacks contentment because Dhyana and Samadhi are the state of deep contentment. In short, you will satisfy all the requirements that are asked of you in the yoga process naturally, even if you don't know about them. Every move you make will be in a total compliance with the laws of nature.

State of Dhyana and Samadhi

To know the space very clearly, start with the preparation exercises shown in Chapter 9. Then do all the Qi-gong exercises with no expectations. Let your arms move like you are touching someone you love. The breathing exercise without expectation is extremely powerful. These techniques will bring you to your center and you will start to feel the state of oneness, the state of Dhyana and Samadhi within and all around you. When you are in the present moment and undisturbed, you are in this state. Once you know this space, you will find that you can come to it in different ways. As this relationship develops, you will crave it like a mother craves her firstborn child or a lover craves his or her beloved. Then you are creating a reference between your personality and the universal consciousness that will be very hard to break, and this reference will always keep you connected. You will become spiritual (or spirit-like). Whenever you move away from it, you will feel a deep pain of separation and be pulled right back into it. Whenever you are in it, you will be in ecstasy or bliss. Then there will be no need to study the rules, commandments, Yamas and Niyamas because they will have become a way of life.

Once you know this space, your asana and Qi-gong practice will become your time to connect and merge into the universal consciousness. You will find that your ego and process of mind has disappeared and so has all the stress of life. In this state you have no fear of anything including death. You will have become totally liberated into a state of Moksha or Samadhi.

Bibliography

Ayurveda
1) The Textbook of Ayurveda: Fundamental Principles by Dr. Vasant Lad.

2) The Complete Book of Ayurvedic Home Remedies by Dr. Vasant Lad.

3) The Yoga of Herbs: An Ayurvedic Guide To Herbal Medicine by Dr. Frawley & Dr. Vasant Lad.

4) Secrets of the Pulse: The Ancient Art of Ayurvedic Pulse Diagnosis by Dr. Vasant Lad.

5) The Ayurveda Encyclopedia by Swami Sada Shiva Thirtha.

Anatomy and Physiology
6) Atlas of Human Anatomy by Frank Netter, M.D. Second Edition, Novartis.

7) Interactive Atlas of Human Anatomy by Frank Netter, M.D.

8) The Human Brain by John Nolte Ph.D.

9) The Melatonin Miracle: Nature's Age-Reversing, Disease-Fighting, Sex-Enhancing Harmone by Walter Pierpaoli.

Yoga
10) Light on Yoga by B. K. S. Iyengar.

11) Light on The Yoga Sutras of Patanjali by B. K. S. Iyengar.

12) Yoga The Method of Re-integration by Alain Danielou.

Qi-Gong
13) Qigong: The Secret of Youth by Dr. Yang, Jwing-Ming. www.YMAA.com.

14) The Root of Chinese Qigong by Dr. Yang, Jwing-Ming. www.YMAA.com.

15) Eight simple Qigong exercises for health by Dr. Yang, Jwing-Ming. www.YMAA.com.

Meditation
16) Enlightenment the Only Revolution: Talks on Astavakras Maha Geeta by Osho. www.Osho.com.

17) An Autobiography of a Spiritually Incorrect Mystic by Osho. www.Osho.com.

18) Meditation: First and Last Freedom by Osho. www.Osho.com.

19) Tao Te Ching by Lao Tsu, Translated by Gia-Fu Feng & Jane English.

Ayurvedic Herbs website
www.garrysun.com

www.bazarofindia.com

Video
The Tibetan Book of the Dead by Wellspring Media. www.wellmedia.com. Baraka. www.Amazon.com.

Meetings with Remarkable Men: Life of George Gurdjieff. www.Amazon.com.

Music
Chuang Tsu's Dream by Anand Milarepa. www.oneskymusic.com

Laughter of the Buddhas by Anand Milarepa. www.oneskymusic.com.

Dakini Lounge by Prem Joshua. www.premjoshua.com.

Sattva by Manish Vyas. www.Manishvyas.com.

Blowing Zen by Devakant. www.devakant.com.

Inside Is Forever by Devakant. www.devakant.com.

Scientific Publications
Salivary Gland References Mathison R.D., Befus, A.D., & Davison, J.S. 1997. A novel submandibular gland peptide protects against endotoxic and anaphylactic shock. American Journal of. Physiology 273: R1017-R1023.

Mathison R.D., Davison J.S., & Befus A.D. 1994. The cervical sympathetic trunk-submandibular gland axis in the regulation of inflammatory responses. Advances in Psychoneuroimmunology (eds. I. Berczi. J Szelenyi) Plenum Press, pp. 303-315.

Mathison R.D., Davison J.S., & Befus A.D. 1994. Neuroendocrine regulation of inflammation and tissue repair by submandibular gland factors. Immunology Today 15: 527-532.

Mathison R.D., Mai J., & Davison J.S. 1995. Endotoxin-induced hypotension exhibits seasonal variation: A role for submandibular glands? Proc West Pharmacol Soc 38: 21-23.

Mathison R.D. 1995. The Submandibular Glands: a role in homeostasis and allostasis. Biomedical Reviews 4: 61-69.

Befus, A.D., Davison J.S., & Mathison R.D. 1997. A peptide from submandibular glands modulates inflammatory responses. Int Arch Allergy Immunol 113: 337-338.

Mathison R.D., Befus A.D., & Davison J.S. 1997. Reduction in cardiovascular anaphylaxis by Submandibular Gland Peptide-T (SGP-T). Proc West Pharmacol Soc 40: 73-74.

Mathison R.D., Malkinson T., Cooper K.E., & Davison J.S. 1997. Submandibular glands: Novel structures participating in thermoregulatory responses. Canadian Journal of Physio Pharmacol 75: 407-413, 1997.

Mathison R.D., Befus A.D., & Davison J.S. 1997. A novel submandibular gland peptide protects against endotoxin-induced hypotension. American Journal of Physiology 273: R1017-R1023.

Mathison R.D., Davison J.S., & Moore G. 1997. Submandibular gland peptide-T (SGP-T): Modulation of endotoxic and anaphylactic shock. Drug Discovery Res 42: 164-171.

Nkemdirim M., Kubera M., & Mathison, R.D. 1998. Modulation of neutrophil activity by submandibular gland peptide-T (SGP-T). Pol J Pharmacol 50: 417-424.

Mathison R.D., Kubera M., & Davison J.S. 1999. Submandibular Gland Peptide-T (SGP-T) modulates ventricular function in response to intravenous endotoxin. Pol J Pharmacol 51: 331-339.

Rougeot C., Rosinski-Chupin I., Mathison R.D., & Rougeon F. 2000. Rodent submandibular gland peptide hormones and other biologically active peptides. Peptides 21: 443-455.

Tan D., Rougeot C., Davison J.S., & Mathison R.D. 2000. The carboxamide feG(NH2) inhibits endotoxin perturbation of intestinal motility. Eur Jour of Pharmacol 409: 203-205.

Mathison R.D., Lo P., Tan D., Scott B., Befus D., & Davison J.S. 2001. The tripeptide FEG and its analogue feG reduce endotoxin provoked perturbation of intestinal motility and inflammation.

Neurogastroenterology & Motility 13: 599-603.

Salim Yusuf, Steven Hawken, Stephanie Ôunpuu, Tony Dans, Alvaro Avezum, Fernando Lanas, Matthew McQueen, Andrzej Budaj, Prem Pais, John Varigos, Liu Lisheng. Effect of potentially modifiable risk factors associated with myocardial infarction in 52 countries (the INTERHEART study): case-control study. The Lancet volume 364 Issue 9438 Page 937. www.thelancet.com.

Black P.H., & Garbutt L.D. January 2002. Stress, inflammation and cardiovascular disease. Journal of Psychosomatic Research vol. 52, iss. 1, pp. 1-23.

Cole-King A., & Gordon Harding K. 2001. Psychological factors and delayed healing in chronic wounds. Psychosomatic Medince 63: 216-220

Pickering, T. 1999. Cardiovascular pathways: Socioeconomic status and stress effects on hypertension and cardiovascular function. Annals of the New York Academy of Sciences 896: 262-277.

Von Kanel, R., Mills, P.J., Fainman, C., & Dimsdale, J.E. 2001. Effects of psychological stress and psychiatric disorders on blood coagulation and fibrinolysis: A biobehavioral pathway to coronary artery disease? Psychosomatic Medicine 63: 531-544.

Cohen, S., Hamrick, N., Rodriguez, M.S., Feldman, P.J., Rabin, B.S., & Manuck. The stability of and intercorrelations among cardiovascular, immune, endocrine, and psychological reactivity. Annals of Behavioral Medicine 22, 171-179.

Malek, A.M., Alper, S.L., & Izumo, S. 1999. Hemodynamic shear stress and its role in atherosclerosis. JAMA 282, 2035-2042.

Kaplan, J.R., & Manuck, S.B. 1999. Status, stress, and atherosclerosis: The role of environment and individual behavior. Annals of the New York Academy of Sciences 896, 145-161.

McCabe, P.M., Schneiderman, N., Field, T.M. et al. (eds.), Stress, Coping, and Disease. Hillsdale, N.J. Lawrence Erlbaum Associates. pp. 51-72.

Cohen, S., Doyle, W.J., & Skoner, D.P. 1999. Psychological stress, cytokine production, and severity of upper respiratory illness. Psychosomatic Medicine 61, 175-180.

Guyton, A.C., Hall, J.E. 2000. Textbook of Medical Physiology, 10th ed. Philadelphia, WB Saunders Co. Chapter on Hemostasis and blood coagulation.*

Markovitz, J.H., & Matthews, K.A. 1991. Platelets and coronary heart disease: Potential psychophysiologic mechanisms.

Psychosomatic Medicine 53, 643-668.

Malkoff, S.B., Muldoon, M.F., Zeigler, Z.R., & Manuck, S.B. 1993. Blood platelet responsivity to acute mental stress. Psychosomatic Medicine 55 477-482.

Nemeroff, C.B., & Musselman, D.L. 2000. Are platelets the link between `depression and ischemic heart disease? American Heart Journal 140, S57-S62.

Camacho, A., & Dimsdale, J.E. 2000. Platelets and psychiatry: Lessons learned from old and new studies. Psychosomatic Medicine 62, 326-336.

Pickering, T.G. 1997. The effects of environmental and lifestyle factors on blood pressure and the intermediary role of the sympathetic nervous system. Journal of Human Hypertension 11 (Supp. 1), S9-S18.

Rutledge, T., & Hogan, B.E. 2002. A quantitative review of prospective evidence linking psychological factors with hypertension development. Psychosomatic Medicine 64, 758-766.

Schnall, P.L., Schwartz, J.E., Landsbergis, P.A., Warren, K., & Pickering, T.G. 1998. A longitudinal study of job strain and ambulatory blood pressure: Results from a three-year follow-up. Psychosomatic Medicine 60, 697-706.

Lipsky, S.I., Pickering, T.G., & Gerin, W. 2002. World Trade Center disaster effect on blood pressure. Blood Pressure Monitoring 7, 249.

Schneider, M.P., Klingbeil, A.U., Schlaich, M.P., Langenfeld, M.R., Veelken, R., & Schmieder, R.E. 2001. Impaired sodium excretion during mental stress in mild essential hypertension. Hypertension 37, 923-927.

Reaven, G.M., Lithell, H., & Landsberg, L. 1996. Mechanisms of disease: Hypertension and associated metabolic abnormalities---the role of insulin resistance and the sympathoadrenal system. New England Journal of Medicine 334, 374-381.

Bjorntorp, P. 2001. Do stress reactions cause abdominal obesity and comorbidities? Obesity Reviews 2, 73-86.

Brunner, E.J., Hemingway, H., Walker, B.R., Page, M., et al. 2002. Adrenocortical, autonomic, and inflammatory causes of the metabolic syndrome: Nested case-control study. Circulation 106, 2659-2665.

Vitaliano, P.P., Scanlan, J.M., Zhang, J., Savage, M.V., Hirsch, I.B., & Siegler, I.C. 2002. A path model of chronic stress, the metabolic syndrome, and coronary heartdisease. Psychosomatic Medicine 64, 418-435.

Sakkinen, P.A., Wahl, P., Cushman, M., et al. 2000. Clustering of procoagulation, inflammation, and fibrinolysis variables with metabolic factors in insulin resistance syndrome. American Journal of Epidemiology 152: 897-907.

Epel, E.S., McEwen, B., Seeman, T., Matthews, K., Castellazzo, G., Brownell, K.D., Bell, J., & Ickovics, J.R. 2000. Stress and body shape: Stress-induced cortisol secretion is consistently greater among women with central fat. Psychosomatic Medicine 62: 623-632.

Krantz, D.S., Kop, W.J., Santiago, H.T., & Gottdiener, J.S. 1996. Mental stress as a trigger of myocardial ischemia and infarction. Cardiology Clinics 14:271-287.

Muller, J.E. 1999. Circadian variation and triggering of acute coronary events. American Heart Journal 137, S1-S8.

Verrier, R.L., & Mittleman, M.A. 1996. Life threatening cardiovascular consequences of anger in patients with CHD. Cardiology Clinics 14, 289-307.*

Sheps, D.S. et al. 2002. Mental stress-induced ischemia and all-cause mortality in patients with coronary artery disease: Results from the Psychophysiological Investigations of Myocardial Ischemia Study. Circulation 105, 1780-1784.

Lampert, R., Joska, T., Burg, M.M., Batsford, W.P., McPherson, C.A., & Jain, D. 2002. Emotional and physical precipitants of ventricular arrhythmia. Circulation 106, 1800-1805.

Kamarck, T., & Jennings, J.R. 1991. Biobehavioral factors in sudden cardiac death. Psychological Bulletin 109, 42-75.

Blumenthal, J.A., Sherwood, A., Gullette, E.C.D., Georgiades, A., & Tweedy, D. 2002. Biobehavioral approaches to the treatment of essential hypertension. Journal of Consulting and Clinical Psychology 70, 569-589.

Surwit, R.S., van Tilburg, M., Zucker, N., McCaskill, C.C., Parekh, P., Feinglos, M.N., Edwards, C.L., Williams, P., & Lane, J.D. 2002. Stress management improves long-term glycemic control in Type 2 diabetes. Diabetes Care 25, 30-34.

Castillo-Richmond, A., Schneider, R.H., Alexander, C.N., Cook, R., Myers, H., Nidich, S., Haney, C., Rainforth, M., & Salerno, J. 2000. Effects of stress reduction on carotid atherosclerosis in hypertensive African Americans. Stroke 31, 568-573.

Castillo-Richmond, A., Payne, K., Clark, E.T., & Rainforth, M. 2002. Effect of a multi-modality natural medicine program on carotid atherosclerosis in older subjects: A pilot trial of Maharishi Vedic Medicine. American Journal of Cardiology 89, 952-958.

Blumenthal, J.A., Babyak, M., Wei, J., O'Connor, C., Waugh, R., Eisenstein, E., Mark, D., Sherwood, A., Woodley, P.S., Irwin, R.J., & Reed, G. 2002. Usefulness of psychosocial treatment of mental stress-induced myocardial ischemia in men. American Journal of Cardiology 8.